COLOR ATLAS
OF
Ophthalmological Diagnosis

M. A. BEDFORD
F.R.C.S.
Consultant Eye Surgeon,
St. Bartholomew's Hospital
and
Moorfields Eye Hospital, London, E.C.1

YEAR BOOK MEDICAL PUBLISHERS, INC.
35 E. WACKER DRIVE–CHICAGO

Books in this series already published
Color Atlas of General Pathology
Color Atlas of Oro-Facial Diseases
Color Atlas of Ophthalmological Diagnosis
Color Atlas of Renal Diseases
Color Atlas of Venereology
Color Atlas of Dermatology
⁻ *Color Atlas of Infectious Diseases*
⁻ *Color Atlas of Ear, Nose & Throat Diagnosis*
Color Atlas of Rheumatology
Color Atlas of Microbiology
Color Atlas of Forensic Pathology
Color Atlas of Pediatrics
Color Atlas of Histology
⁻ *Color Atlas of General Surgical Diagnosis*
Color Atlas of Physical Signs in General Medicine
Color Atlas of Tropical Medicine and Parasitology
Color Atlas of Human Anatomy
Color Atlas of Cardiac Pathology
Color Atlas of Histological Staining Techniques
Atlas of Cardiology, ECG's and Chest X-Rays

Some further titles now in preparation
Color Atlas of Neuropathology
Color Atlas of Oral Anatomy
Color Atlas of Oral Medicine
Color Atlas of Gynecological Surgery (6 volumes)
Color Atlas of Tumors of the Eye
Color Atlas of Liver Diseases
Color Atlas of Periodontology
Color Atlas of Diabetes Mellitus

Contents

Introduction

THIS WORK is intended to be an atlas, not a textbook. No attempt is made to cover the whole field of ophthalmology. The book is aimed at the hard-pressed undergraduate or family doctor who has not the time (or the inclination) to delve deeply into a textbook containing optical theory and obscure pathological conditions surrounded by complicated ocular terms unlike any others in the rest of medicine.

In the first chapter emphasis is placed on a practical examination which is described step by step and which can be carried out with a minimum of simple instrumentation by someone not necessarily skilled in ophthalmology. In addition there are short descriptions of diagnostic instruments an eye surgeon may use.

This is followed by chapters dealing with the evaluation of common clinical patterns that the non-ophthalmologist may be confronted with; that is, the red eye; loss of vision in an apparently normal looking white eye; eye injuries, and so on. In each of these chapters an attempt is made to show how the diagnosis can be made by employing the method of examination previously described.

It is hoped that this atlas may help the average medical man to sort out ocular problems which might well otherwise defeat him.

Part 1

Methods of examination

1. Estimation of the Visual Acuity: Figs. 1 & 2

2. Examination of the Outside of the Eye: Figs. 3–9

3. Examination of the Inside of the Eye: Figs. 10–15

Other tests not used routinely

(A) Assessment of Intra-ocular Pressure:
Figs. 17–19

(B) Assessment of Visual Fields: Figs. 21–25

METHODS OF EXAMINATION

Fig. 1. When confronted with a patient complaining of an ocular disorder of any sort, the first point to establish is: what can the patient actually see? This is estimated with the well known Snellen test chart which should be used at a distance of 6 metres from the patient; this "6" is the top number of the fraction 6/6; being the normal visual acuity. On the figure opposite, this is the ability to read the third line from the bottom. The lowest two lines are necessary because very often the patient's visual acuity can be better than normal, *i.e.* 6/5 (second line from the bottom) or 6/4 (being the bottom line). The reasoning behind this chart is that, taking the top letter, the normal person can see this at 60 metres as it subtends ten times the angle of the letters on the 6/6 line. Similarly, a normal person can see the second line *i.e.* "O E" at 36 metres and underneath that 24, 18, 12 and 9 metres. If testing at 6 metres and the patient can see only the second line from the top ("O E") the vision is thus 6/36. There are several points to bear in mind when testing the visual acuity; do not waste time doing binocular visual acuity, but test one eye at a time and always test the eye the patient is not complaining about first as this can be a very useful control.

The approximate equivalents to Snellen's notation in feet and in the decimal system are:—

Snellen's notation		Decimal notation
Metres	Feet	
6/6	20/20	1·0
6/9	20/30	0·7
6/12	20/40	0·5
6/18	20/60	0·3
6/24	20/80	0·25
6/60	20/200	0·1

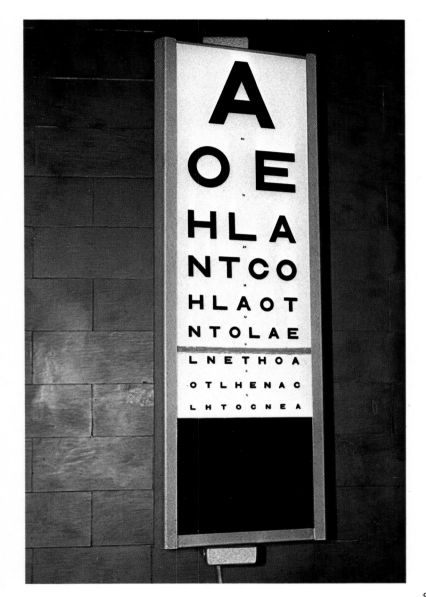

9

Fig. 2. Always use an opaque card to occlude the other eye. If you use your own hand or the patient's hand there may be small gaps between the fingers, through which the patient may sometimes look, thus giving a false reading. The card can be easily moved across to the other eye; there is thus no doubt as to the separate visual acuity of each eye. Naturally, the tests should be done with the patient wearing his distance glasses or bifocals. This is a point well worth remembering, for to save time the patient, knowing that he is to see the doctor about his eyes, will tend to remove his glasses before coming in for the examination.

Fig. 3. Next consider the examination proper; taking it in a logical order. Firstly, examine the outside of the eye. This is best done by using an ordinary hand light and holding up the upper lid as shown. Points to be noticed are: Is the eye white or red? Are the pupils reacting normally? Is there a nice bright corneal reflex? This last is a sight which pleases all eye surgeons, for it proves that the essential transparent window of the eye – the cornea – is probably normal, if the highlight shown by the reflection of the examiner's hand light is bright and clearly defined.

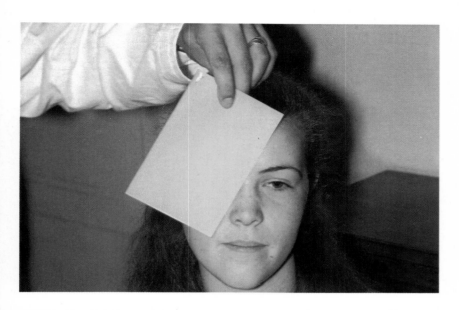

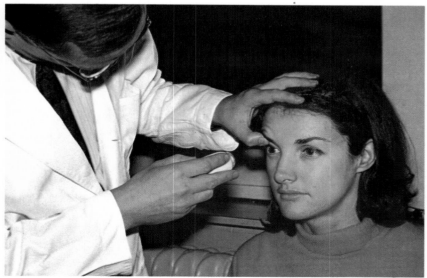

Figs. 4 & 4a. The patient should be instructed to look to the right, to the left, up and down. Both eyes should be examined in this way. It is impossible to see the deep aspect of the upper lid without a further manoeuvre termed "eversion" (Fig. 5).

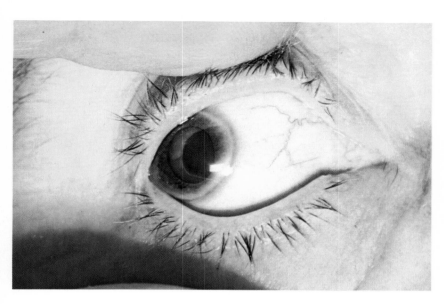

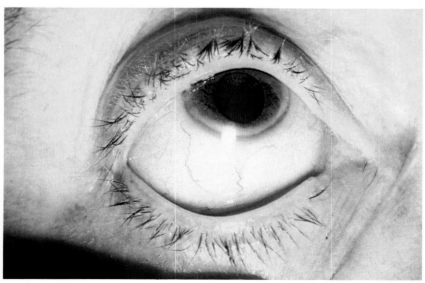

Fig. 5. It may be necessary to evert the upper lid, particularly if the patient is complaining of, say, a foreign body which has not so far become apparent in the routine examination. The best method is to stand behind the patient as shown. When everting the right upper lid, the doctor should pull the lid out with his right hand, then turn the lid over the index finger of his left hand.

Fig. 6. The lid is now everted and any foreign body present is easily removed. Such movements, of course, should be reversed for the eversion of the left upper lid. If the foreign body has been present for some time, whenever the patient has blinked a linear corneal ulcer will have been formed. These ulcers may be very severe; their size may be estimated by applying fluorescein (**Fig. 7**).

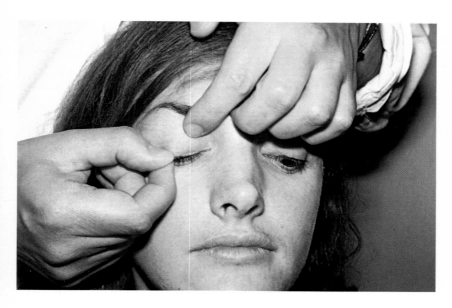

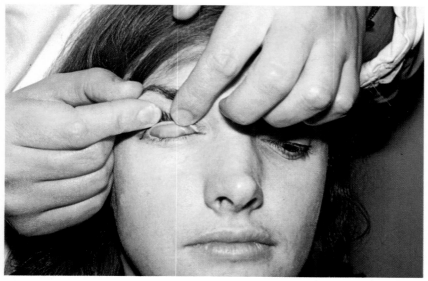

Fig. 7. The application of fluorescein is essential in making the diagnosis of loss of epithelium on a transparent structure like the cornea, for it is impossible to see with the naked eye. The classical form of fluorescein as eye drops can be seen in the bottle in the photograph, the excess being removed from the cornea by saline drops. There are certain shortcomings to this because the fluorescein in eye drops may grow pseudomonas pyocyneus after a period of some weeks. It is unfair to expect the average practitioner to change his drops every so often to prevent this deterioration, so there are two alternatives. On the left there is a small holder containing many pieces of filter paper with fluorescein impregnated at one end. These are probably ideal, for they will last for many months. All that is needed is to tear off a small piece of filter paper and rub it once or twice in the lower fornix; then ask the patient to blink — and a minute trace of fluorescein will cover the whole of the outside of the eye; an ulcer if present, will be picked out as a brilliant green area. **(Fig. 7a).** The other alternative is the plastic prepacked fluorescein droppers which are sterile and used only once. These are theoretically ideal, but are very expensive; their cost probably precludes their routine use.

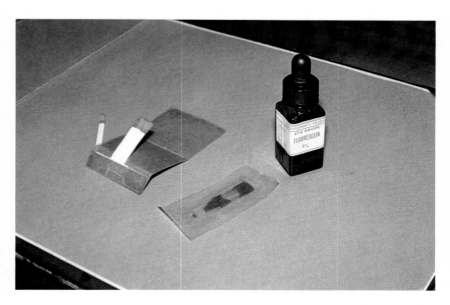

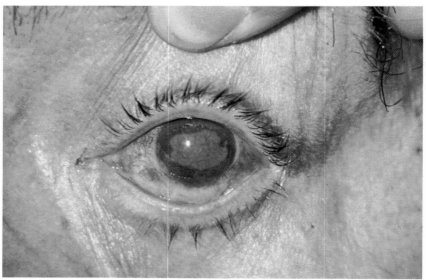

Fig. 8. We have seen from the foregoing exposition how the general practitioner, with his limited resources, may examine the outside of the eye. However, the eye surgeon has more sophisticated equipment; he can, for instance, work with the instrument seen here to look at the anterior half of the eye under magnification. This instrument is a slit-lamp, basically a microscope mounted slightly obliquely to a very thin beam of light which can give an optical section of the front half of the eye, as shown in **fig. 9.**

Fig. 9. On the left is the curved beam of light striking the cornea and passing over towards the right into the anterior chamber of the eye, striking the iris and the lens. In the anterior chamber are some white spots which are aggregations of cells denoting inflammatory pathology inside the eye. This instrument is essential in the management of all serious eye diseases.

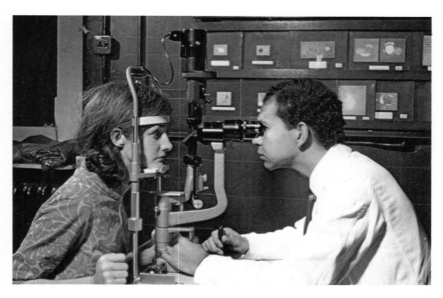

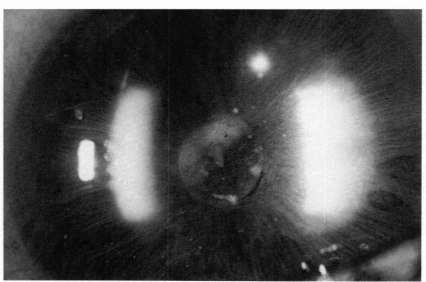

19

Fig. 10. The inside of the eye should now be examined with the ophthalmoscope. Valuable information however may be found by keeping a foot away from the patient and looking through the ophthalmoscope as shown here. Note that the clinician is examining the **right** eye of the patient, using his **right** eye with the ophthalmoscope in his **right** hand.

Fig. 11. This view may be seen through the ophthalmoscope employing this manoeuvre in the normal eye. There is the normal **"red reflex"** as it is termed – and remember that it is red because the light is being reflected back from the choroid, the overlying retina being virtually transparent. It means that (1) there must be transparent media in front of the retina and (2) that the retina is adposed to the choroid. Thus any loss of the red reflex means that there is either (a) an opacity in the media preventing the light from going through or (b) the retina is not against the choroid and is out of position. In terms of pathology there is one of three conditions: a cataract, a vitreous haemorrhage or a retinal detachment.

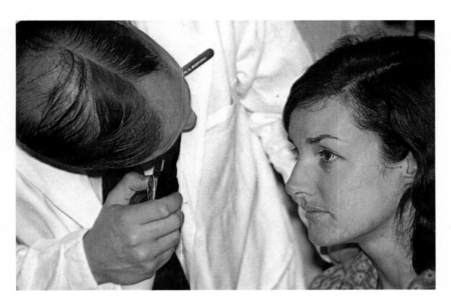

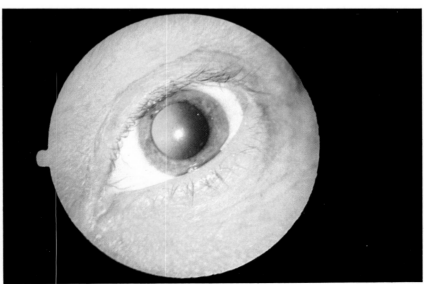

Fig. 12. Note that there is no red reflex, but a rather characteristic greyness which suggests that there is a total retinal detachment. Such a similar loss of red reflex particularly associated with an opacity which can be seen anteriorly, while using the hand light in the examination of the outside of the eye, would mean that a cataract is present. Having seen the normal red reflex the examiner should then move his head and ophthalmoscope near to the patient – and emphasis is placed on the **nearness**.

Fig. 13. Notice that the examiner's forehead is actually touching the patient's forehead. This is logical – to look at the view from a window, one gets as close to the window as possible. There is no other way of examining the inside of the eye properly than to get as **close as possible**, and for this reason the examiner uses his **right** eye with the ophthalmoscope in his **right** hand when looking at the **right** eye of the patient and reverses all these manoeuvres when examining the left eye. It is impossible to examine a patient's fundus if both the examiner and the patient are standing up: one cannot get close enough.

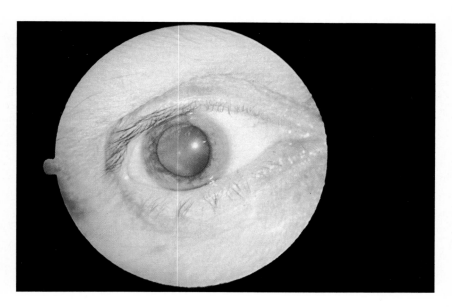

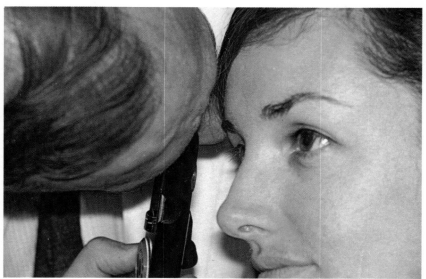

Fig. 14. The view of the normal fundus as seen with the ophthalmoscope. The following points should be noted:

1. **The disc** – its colour, its cup and its margins. Note the healthy pink colour, the central white depression which is the cup and the well defined margins.

2. **The vessels** – note their calibre and their crossing, then look at the general **background** colour of the fundus, which may vary and should be correlated with the colouring and race of the patient.

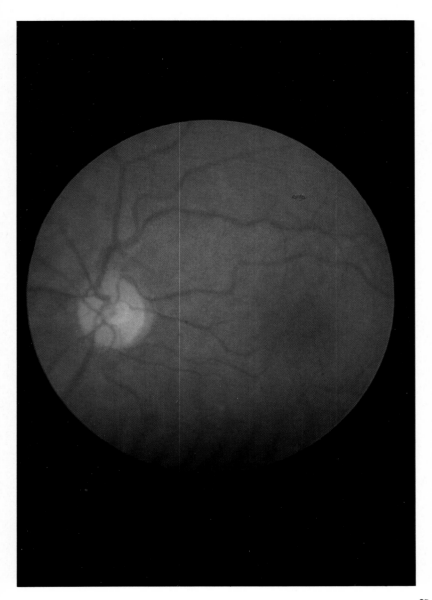

Fig. 15. A dark fundus which may be seen in a negro person. The fine white lines are light reflections from the retinal fibres.

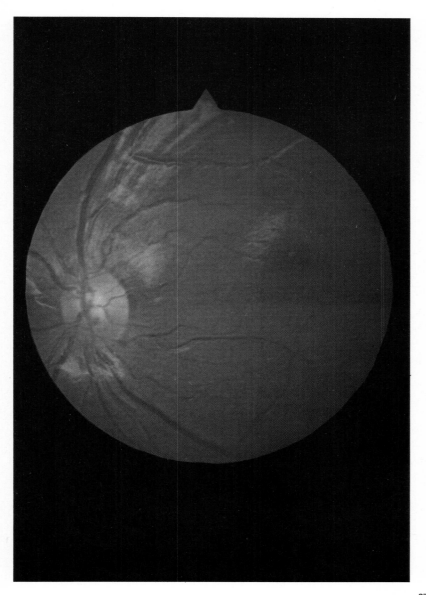

27

Fig. 16. A typical myopic albinoid fundus showing the myopic "crescent" around the disc and the general thinning of the retina and choroid, the choroidal vessels showing through as flat ribbons because of the small amount of pigment epithelium present beneath the retina. Through the undilated pupil only the disc and paramacular area may be seen and at this point if one's suspicions are aroused the pupils may be dilated. A short-acting mydriatic (pupil-dilating) drop should be used such as Cyclopentolate, Tropicamide or Hyoscine — never Atropine, for its action lasts for ten to fourteen days.

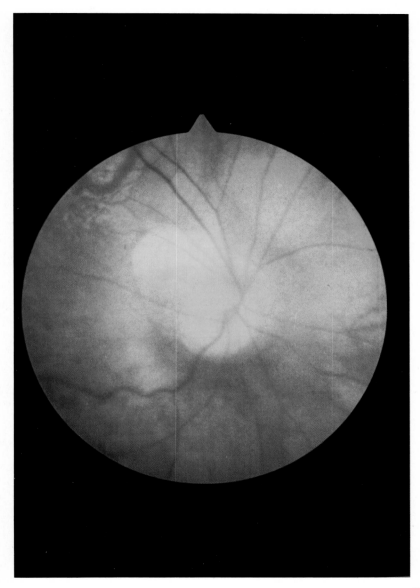

Fig. 17. If necessary and particularly if the diagnostic problem of acute glaucoma has been raised, it will be essential to assess the intra-ocular pressure. This is done by **digital palpation** as can be seen here. Note that both hands rest on the patient's forehead; one would assess the normal eye first and then the eye under suspicion. Most examiners will probably never pick up the slight elevation in both eyes in chronic simple glaucoma **(figs. 55 & 56),** but relatively unskilled observers can easily pick up the very high pressure characteristics of an acute glaucoma **(figs. 33 to 35)** in one eye. A discrepancy is only too obvious if the normal eye is palpated first.

Fig. 18. The classical way of measuring the intra-ocular pressure as practised in eye hospitals is with the **Schiøtz tonometer.** Below can be seen a small plunger about to rest on the anaesthetised cornea; obviously the degree that the plunger moves down governs the sweep of the pointer above. This is not very accurate and another technique is used in most modern eye departments, as seen in **fig. 19.**

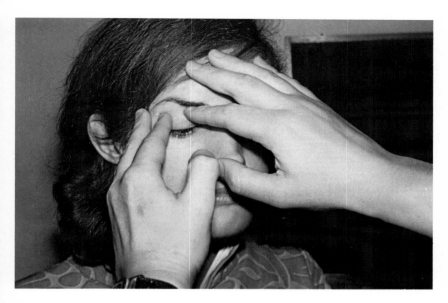

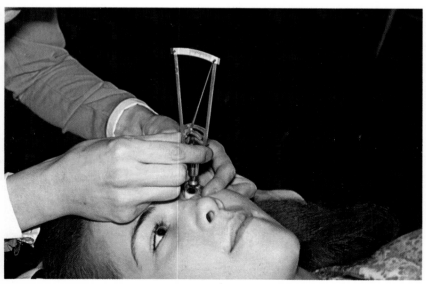

Fig. 19. This is a little prism mounted on the slit-lamp which is rested delicately on the front of the cornea. The amount of force used to produce a standard deformation is measured and this gives an index of the pressure **(applanation tonometry).** This is probably the most accurate method of measuring the intra-ocular pressure at present.

Fig. 20. If necessary the state of the tear passages may be assessed by syringing them. The patient may feel the water running into his nose if the passages are clear. This is a manoeuvre that can be done by medical practitioners but it is time-consuming, needs a special cannula, and in most cases is probably best done by the surgeon at hospital.

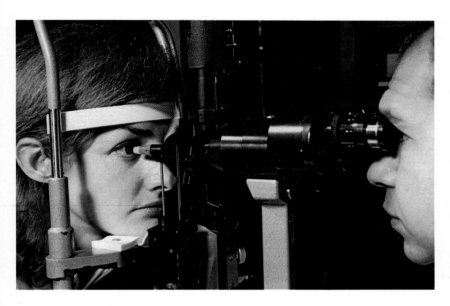

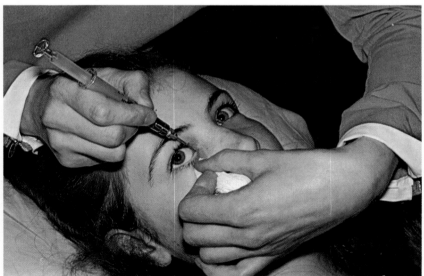

Fig. 21. If necessary, the other aspect of visual function, *i.e.* the visual fields, may be assessed. These need not be estimated in every case as they are time-consuming, but should be reserved for the problem of the patient who has had difficulty in seeing with optimum spectacle lenses and where there is no ocular pathology yet noted in the examination, or perhaps a suspicion of optic atrophy has been seen with the ophthalmoscope. The fields are easily done by **confrontation** but note that the examiner's hand is covering the eye which is not being examined, and the patient's other eye is being fixed by the examiner's opposite eye to make sure the point of fixation does not move. Note also that as the examiner is comparing the patient's visual field with his own – the examiner's hand is exactly halfway between them. Such a method of examination is very rough; should a defect be picked up it should be examined in detail on a machine such as that seen in the next figure.

Fig. 22. The patient is maintaining her gaze on the central white spot while a nurse is rotating a handle at the back of the machine which moves the peripheral white spot; as this moves inwards the patient signifies when she first sees it.

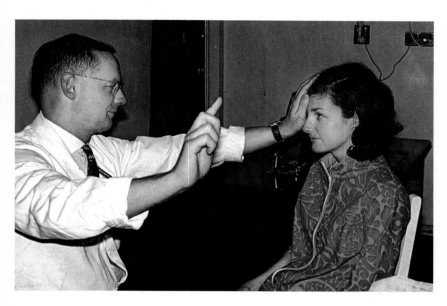

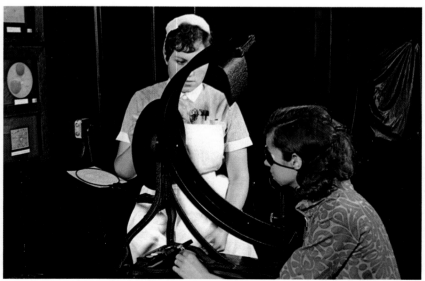

Fig. 23. There is a metal spike on the back of the machine which is geared to move with the white spot actuated by the nurse who merely moves the card up and punches a hole in it at the appropriate moment.

Fig. 24. The **peripheral field** here seen on the right is of course of one eye and is restricted above and nasally. This is the right peripheral field and the restrictions are due to the brow and nose. The defect seen, as marked by red ink, is a temporal hemianopia and if present in both eyes would signify a pituitary tumour. Unfortunately pituitary tumours can produce not peripheral field defects, as noted here, but **central field** defects and the larger chart which you can see on the left corresponds to only 30° from the central point of vision. It is a very magnified area of the centre of the peripheral field chart. A field defect can occur just within a few degrees of fixation and can have the same sinister significance as a larger peripheral field defect. This sort of central field scotoma will not be picked up by the perimeter and has to be done in a special way.

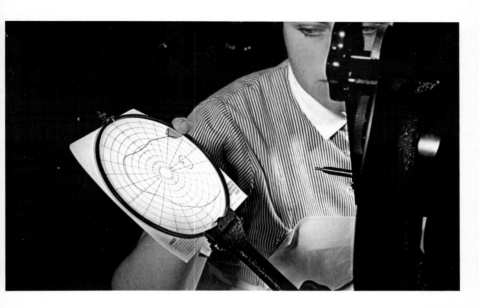

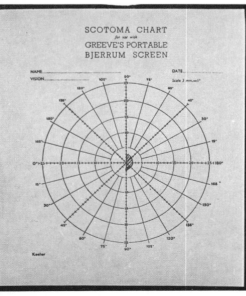

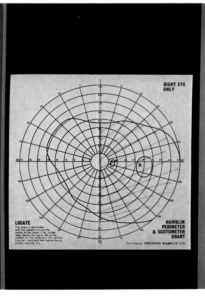

Fig. 25. This shows an examiner dressed in black so as not to distract the patient's fixation. He holds a wand terminating in a white spot and the patient signifies whether he can see it or not as it is moved around. The examiner then places in a series of small pins and maps out the blind spots when present. Such a test is time-consuming and is probably one of the most accurate methods of doing a central visual field.

Although some of the steps here clearly should be undertaken by a special examiner with special equipment, *e.g.* slit-lamp, tonometer, peripheral and central fields, the salient points of the examination can be achieved with three simple instruments:

(1) The **visual acuity chart** to determine the visual function;

(2) The **hand light** to examine the outside of the eye;

(3) The **ophthalmoscope** to examine the inside of the eye.

In the ensuing chapters this method of examination will be emphasised when sorting out the diagnosis of the red eye or loss of vision in a white eye, etc. as it can be easily practised almost anywhere.

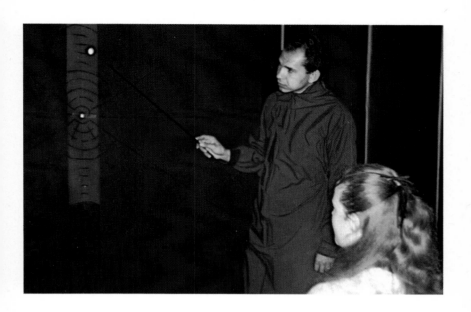

Part 2

The Red Eye

IN THIS CHAPTER we will endeavour to sort out what is probably the most common clinical problem that can be seen by the family doctor – the "red eye". Emphasis will be placed on the method of examination previously described and each colour plate will be discussed as if it is the patient that the doctor is actually examining.

1. Blepharitis   Fig. 26

2. Conjunctivitis   Figs. 27 & 28

3. Iridocyclitis   Figs. 29–32

4. Acute Glaucoma   Figs. 33–35

5. Non-traumatic Corneal Ulcers   Figs. 36–39

These conditions will be diagnosed primarily by examining **the outside of the eye** (figs. 3–9).

Figs. 26 & 26a. This patient is complaining of sore red eyes or red eye-lids which have been present perhaps for some months. He may complain of itching, irritating or soreness, the element of pain being small, the symptoms being more of a trivial nature but very persistent and worrying.

On examination, his visual acuity is normal; the outside of his eye examined with a hand light shows the physical signs seen in the figures, and the inside of the eye is normal on examination with the ophthalmoscope. It will be seen that the eye is white or it may be slightly congested and there is a nice bright corneal reflex, the pupils reacting briskly. The only relevant physical signs are **red and thickened eye-lids** with some **scaling** along the margins. This is termed **blepharitis.** The condition is essentially infective in nature, but there is little point in giving eye drops to be instilled in the conjunctival sac as this is not primarily involved in the pathology. A clue to the precise pathology can be seen on examination of the eye-lashes, when it is noticed that they may be missing or, as in these cases, perhaps deformed and not pointing in their true direction. The infection is thus in the follicle of the lash and any treatment given must be aimed at this site. Useful treatment is to ask the patient to apply an anti-biotic eye ointment by putting it on his little finger and then instructing him to rub it into the roots of his eye-lashes night and morning. This will enable the scales to be removed and for the antibiotic to reach down into the follicles. Treatment may take many weeks or months and in some cases the condition is almost impossible to cure. It is almost always bilateral, but can be asymmetrical.

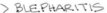
> BLEPHARITIS

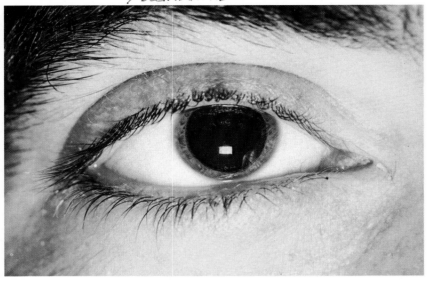

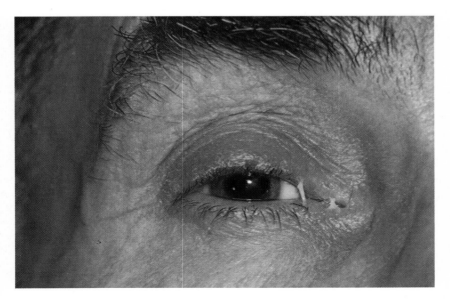

Figs. 27 & 27a. This patient may state that his eyes are sore and red and have been so for several days. On examination, his visual acuity is normal, the outside of his eye shows these physical signs, **congestion being present on the back of the lids and on the membrane reflected upwards from the lower fornix to the limbus** (that is the line of junction where the transparent window of the eye, the cornea, fuses with the white protective sclera and the conjunctiva). There is only one structure continuous on the lid and the globe and that is the conjunctiva, so this is a **conjunctivitis** and classically the congestion is less adjacent to the limbus, for the conjunctiva is thinner there.

Conjunctivitis may be defined as an acute inflammatory condition usually viral or bacterial in nature. In the busy general practice this is of academic importance, for certainly most cases will never be cultured. The classical signs and symptoms are a feeling of **soreness or grittiness**; pain is not usually predominant; the eyes are **red and congested**; it is **bilateral but can be asymmetrical** as one would expect from an infective condition. The visual acuity is of course unaffected, as the essential seeing mechanism of the eye is not involved in the inflammation. However, at times some discharge may collect over the cornea which disturbs vision but this is cleared by blinking and is thus only momentary in nature. One of the classical symptoms is that the patient's eye-lids stick together overnight as of course the secretions dry at the lid margins.

Treatment is vigorous and usually means applications of a suitable antibiotic drop with an antibiotic ointment at night. Should the case not respond in seven to ten days the diagnosis should be reconsidered. **Never make a diagnosis of a monocular conjunctivitis.** In view of the definition stated it presupposes that a monocular conjunctivitis is not infective, *i.e.* it must be secondary to other pathology, that is a missed foreign body, or blocked tear passages, or, what is more likely, it may not be a conjunctivitis at all.

CONJUNCTIVITIS

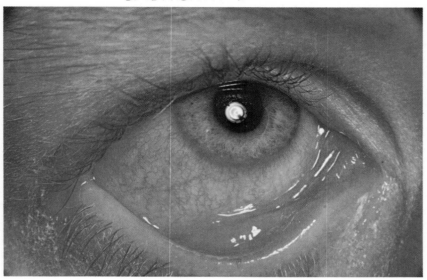

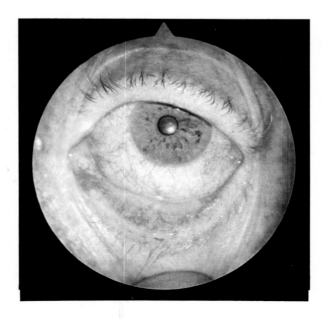

Fig. 28. Occasionally systemic conditions present with a conjunctivitis which does not respond fully to conventional means. Here is the lower conjunctival sac of a patient complaining of a sore red eye which persisted in spite of antibiotic drops. Closer examination reveals a small gelatinous nodule which on biopsy showed the classical appearances of sarcoidosis.

G sarcoid follicles

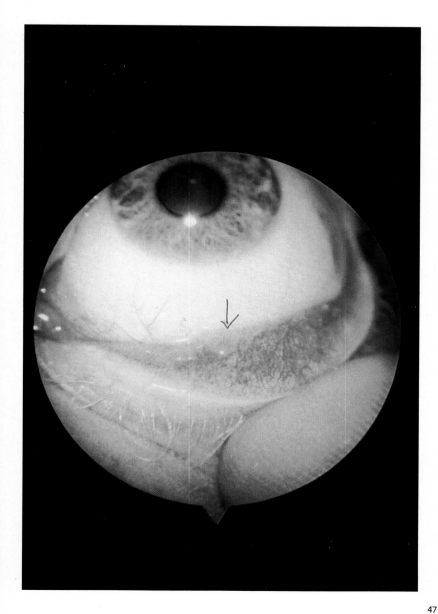

Fig. 29. Note the type of congestion demonstrated by this photograph. **The redness is maximal adjacent to the limbus and grows less** as it spreads to the fornices to the back of the lid. Clearly this is the reverse of the congestion of a conjunctivitis; an eye showing this sort of congestion should be examined with extreme caution as it is highly likely that the essential seeing mechanism inside the eye is involved in an inflammatory process of one sort or another.

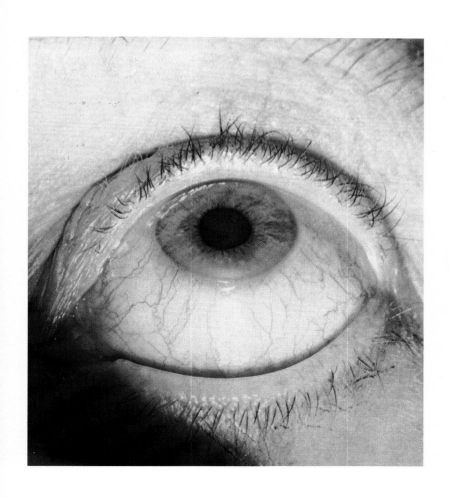

Figs. 30 & 31. This patient complains of a sore red eye with a loss of vision lasting for several days. It may be bilateral but is usually unilateral. On examination the visual acuity shows perhaps a slight loss, it may be 6/18 or 6/12. It is difficult to see the inside of the eye because of the haze situated anteriorly within the globe.

The first point to notice is that the **pupil is irregular** and the general details of the iris are rather hazy. The congestion does **not** involve the back of the lids. The haze must be due to pathology anterior to the iris and there are only two structures situated here. They are *(a)* the outermost transparent cornea and *(b)* the aqueous separating the cornea from the iris. Note that there is a nice bright corneal reflex present showing that the cornea is normal so the essential haze is between the cornea and the iris – that is, the anterior chamber. Correlating this with an acute red eye, this must mean an inflammatory exudate showing that this is a case of an **acute iridocyclitis,** or inflammation of the iris and ciliary body. The physical signs may be built up by applying the principles of inflammation as can be seen in the rest of the body. Clearly there will be swelling and the iris swells in all dimensions, in width and thickness, so that the pupil will be small and slightly sticky because of the inflammatory exudate within it and around it. As it is sticky, the pupillary margin adheres to the lens and sticks in the points seen in the figure which are termed "posterior synechiae" which may become permanent **(fig. 31).**

If the exudate is severe enough the aggregations of cells may be seen as minute white spots in the centre of the pupil (see **fig. 30).** These are classically adherent to the back of the cornea and are termed K.P. or keratic precipitates. The patient is better referred to an eye specialist, as it could be that the condition is not an isolated intra-ocular inflammation but part of a general systemic disease which may require further investigation; *e.g.* a collagen disease; auto-immune disease; some venereal diseases; ankylosing spondylitis; diabetes; Reiter's, etc.

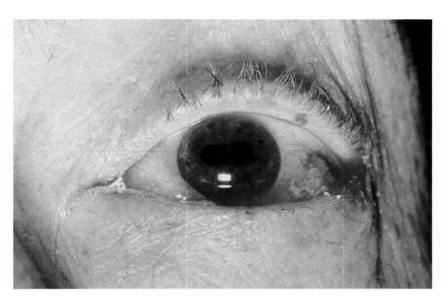

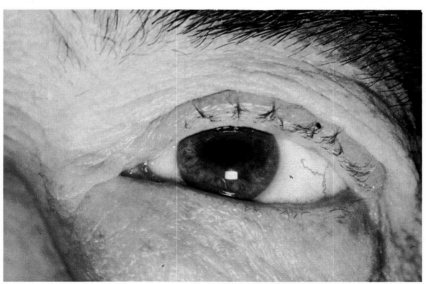

Fig. 32. In early cases if the pupil can be fully dilated the aggregates of cells may be seen against the red reflex of the fundus by using an ophthalmoscope as seen here (or by the slit-lamp used by the eye-surgeon).

In summary then, **acute iridocyclitis** is an inflammatory but not infective process of the iris and ciliary body characterised by a **red eye, visual loss and a small sticky pupil.** Treatment is to dilate the pupil with Atropine, Homatropine or Hyoscine and to suppress the inflammation with either systemic or local steroids.

— RED EYE
— VISUAL LOSS
— SMALL PUPIL
— STICKY PUPIL   —> post - synechiae

℞: ① Dilate pupil
    - Atropine
    - Homatropine
    - Mydriacyl

    ② systemic or local steroids

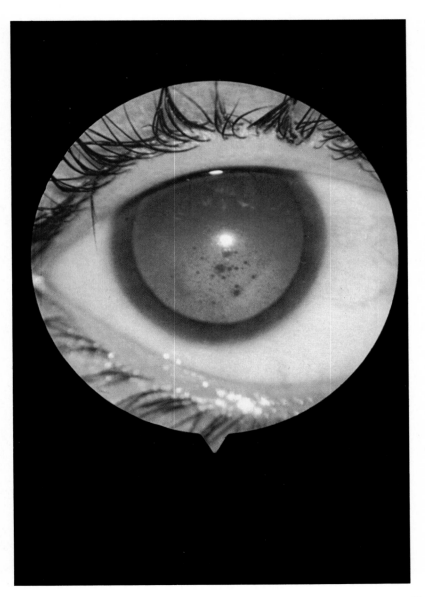

Fig. 33. This patient complains of a sudden severe loss of vision, perhaps preceded by haloes around lights and pain which may be appalling – he may vomit and even collapse. On examination the visual acuity may be less than 6/60 and examination of the outside of his eye shows there is a haze anterior to the iris; because of this haze examination of the inside of the eye with the ophthalmoscope is impossible. The same reasoning should now apply as in the previous case of acute iridocyclitis, when the iris was also obscured by a haze. However, note that in this case the bright corneal reflex is lacking, so the haze must be caused by a disturbance of the cornea. This disturbance is **corneal oedema** and is pathognomonic of an **acute glaucoma** or an acute rise in intra-ocular pressure (the increased pressure forcing fluid into the cornea giving the oedema). Note that because the seeing mechanism of the eye is involved **congestion is limbal** in nature *i.e.* maximal at the junction of the cornea and sclera and conjunctiva. The pressure may rise so high that there may be pressure necrosis of the sphincter and the pupil becomes dilated and fixed.

Fig. 34. A further case of acute glaucoma showing the severe corneal oedema and the classical limbal congestion. Note also that an attempt has been made at surgical treatment by removal of part of the iris.

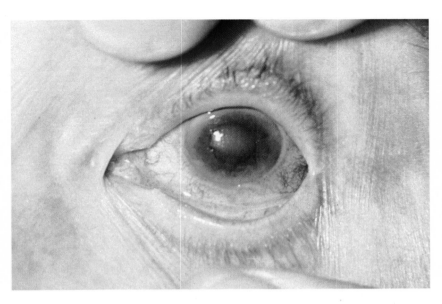

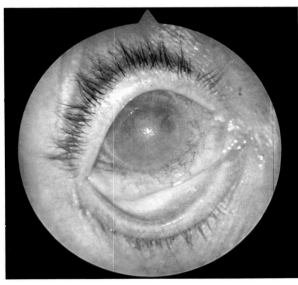

Fig. 35. A diagram showing the flow of aqueous from the ciliary body around the pupillary border, as shown by the red arrow, into the angle. The angle is adjacent to the circular canal of Schlemm which runs around the limbus; the aqueous humour after draining out here passes into the subconjunctival plexus of blood vessels. There is a continuous flow of aqueous and blockage in the angle will give rise to a precipitate increase in the intra-ocular pressure.

Eyes vary in their shape; there can be short fat eyes and long thin eyes. Acute glaucoma appears in rather short fat eyes (hypermetropic or far sighted) where the angles are "crowded" to begin with. As the volume of the iris is constant it can be either long and thin (pupil small) or short and fat (pupil large) and when it is short and fat it may obstruct the angle and cause the intra-ocular pressure to rise. This gives an ophthalmic emergency as the pressure must be reduced as rapidly as possible by giving drops to make the pupil smaller, *e.g.* Pilocarpine and Eserine, thus freeing the angle. All cases should be admitted to hospital, as operation may be needed.

In summary, there is **severe pain and marked visual loss** with **corneal oedema** and classically an **oval, eccentric, dilated pupil.** Treatment is to make the pupil smaller. It must be reiterated that the treatment of acute iridocyclitis and acute glaucoma is exactly opposite.

- severe pain
- marked visual loss
- corneal oedema
- oval, eccentric, dilated pupil

Rx: miotics (make pupil smaller.)

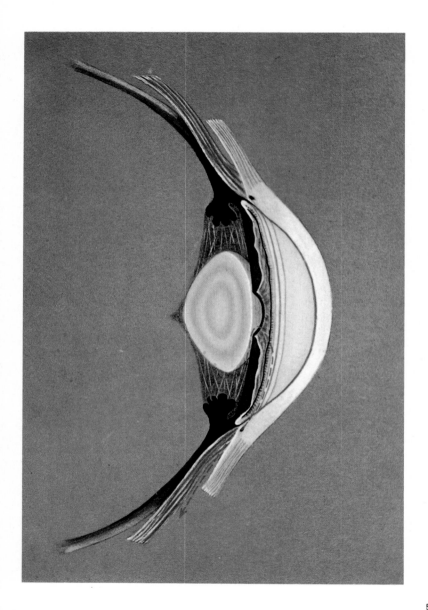

Fig. 36. There is one other condition which may appear as a painful red eye and that is an acute corneal ulcer. There are two forms of corneal ulcers: *(1)* non-traumatic and *(2)* traumatic. The latter will be discussed in a later chapter.

Non-traumatic corneal ulcers are diagnosed by the instillation of fluorescein as described in the methods of examination; the corneal ulcer will then be picked out as a green area of varying dimensions as seen in the figure. The patient complains of a sore, red eye, the visual acuity may be unaffected, and the clue that it is a corneal condition may be given by the fact that there may be varying amounts of blepharospasm and lacrimation. Should this be noted fluorescein should be immediately instilled and the ulcer will be seen, which in this case overlies the pupil.

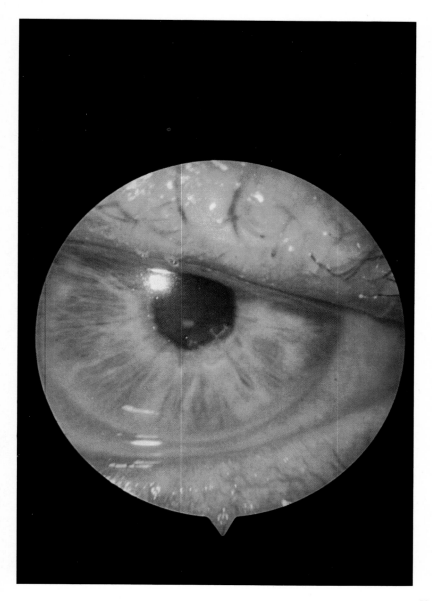

Fig. 37. The fluorescein can be made more obvious by applying a cobalt blue light with the slit-lamp as seen in this figure, demonstrating a non-traumatic corneal ulcer caused by the herpes simplex virus and termed a **dendritic ulcer** as in the previous figure. The treatment of all corneal ulcers is to cover the eye with a pad and bandage, but it is probably best if these common non-traumatic ulcers are referred for specialist attention as they may progress and cause corneal scarring with loss of vision. In no circumstances must these cases be given local steroids as this would facilitate the spread of herpes simplex virus and prevent healing. (See next case, **fig. 38.**)

No steroids in herpes simplex keratitis

Fig. 38. This patient may give a history that she attended for treatment some weeks before with sore red eyes and that she was prescribed eyedrops; her eyes then felt better, now they suddenly feel worse. On examination this characteristic picture is seen: The eye is congested, the white level is pus in the anterior chamber. This is termed an **hypopyon,** and although it may arise spontaneously in some conditions, it should be borne in mind that the patient may previously have been prescribed eye-drops which contained local steroids which would of course facilitate the growth of any organisms. It is dangerous to prescribe local steroids with or without an antibiotic unless adequate slit-lamp serial observation is made. Hypopyon ulcers are extremely serious as the infection has to pass only into the vitreous jelly inside the eye and a pan-ophthalmitis will occur. Occasionally an hypopyon may be seen as part of a systemic collagen disease upset. All cases of hypopyon should be referred for urgent specialist treatment.

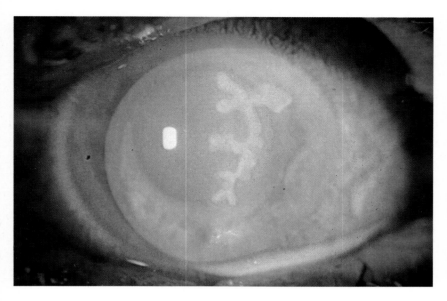

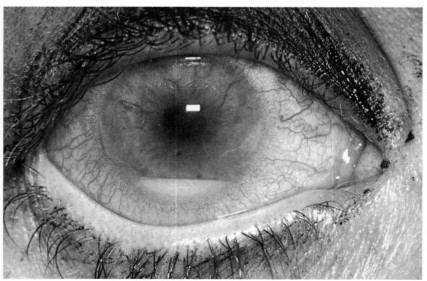

61

Fig. 39. Occasionally a patient may complain of rather odd atypical symptoms with a sore, red eye. A valuable clue may be had by examining the face of the patient, as in this case. This is a case of **herpes zoster ophthalmicus** and such a condition should always be referred for expert treatment, for apart from corneal ulceration, iridocyclitis, glaucoma, optic atrophy and retinal changes the condition may give chronic pain which may last for years.

Although the diagnosis is obvious in this patient, sometimes only a few vesicles may be present on the brow and nose. In all cases of red eyes it is well worth while viewing the patient as a complete person initially before becoming too involved with the local condition.

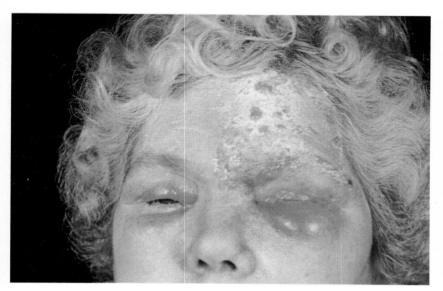

> HERPES ZOSTER OPHTHALMICUS

Part 3

Loss of vision in a White Eye

THERE ARE MANY CAUSES for loss of vision in an apparently normal looking white eye. As the globe looks virtually normal from the outside we have to consider all structures posterior to the iris. The visual changes can be sub-divided into (*1*) gradual loss, and (*2*) sudden loss. Then each of these sub-divisions should be classified further on an anatomical basis, working posteriorly from the lens to the retina, the choroid, optic disc and optic nerves to the chiasm. In all these cases the patient has come to the doctor saying he is not seeing so well and it has come on either suddenly or gradually.

1. GRADUAL
Cataract Figs. 40–45
Retinal Changes
Systemic diseases – Hypertension Figs. 46 & 47;
52–54
Diabetes Fig. 48
Inflammations –Toxoplasmosis Fig. 50
–Syphilis Fig. 51
Papilloedema Figs. 52–54
Optic Nerves
Chronic glaucoma Figs. 55 & 56
Atrophy Fig. 57

2. SUDDEN
Retinal
Vascular –Arterial block Fig. 58
–Venous block Fig. 59
Detachment Figs. 60 & 61

These conditions will be diagnosed primarily by:
1. Estimation of the visual acuity Figs. 1 & 2
2. Examination of the inside of the eye Figs. 10–14

GRADUAL LOSS OF VISION

Fig. 40. This shows a complete opacity of the lens known as a **mature or ripe cataract**. The vision will be less than 6/60. On examination of the outside of the eye the opacity would appear as white. However, with the ophthalmoscope no light would be entering into the eye to be reflected back from the retina and choroid so there would be no red reflex: it would be completely black. This is true of all lens opacities; when looking **at** them they appear white and when attempting to look **through** them they appear black or grey.

Fig. 41 shows a row of minute white flecks concentric with the pupil when they are looked at with the hand light.

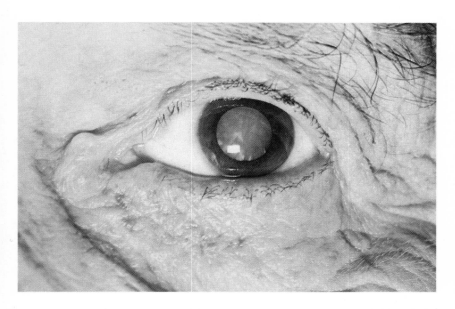

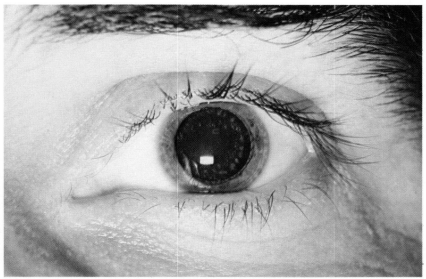

Fig. 42 shows a row of similar opacities which may be seen against the red reflex when using the ophthalmoscope. Cataracts may be classified as *(1)* congenital, *(2)* senile and *(3)* acquired. The third group (acquired) is very large as lens opacities may be considered as interferences in the lens metabolism of any sort, *e.g.* radiation, drugs, injury, etc. The opacity in the lens will develop only while the interference with metabolism is occurring, thus the localisation of the lens opacity and its shape may give a valuable clue as to the cause of the cataract.

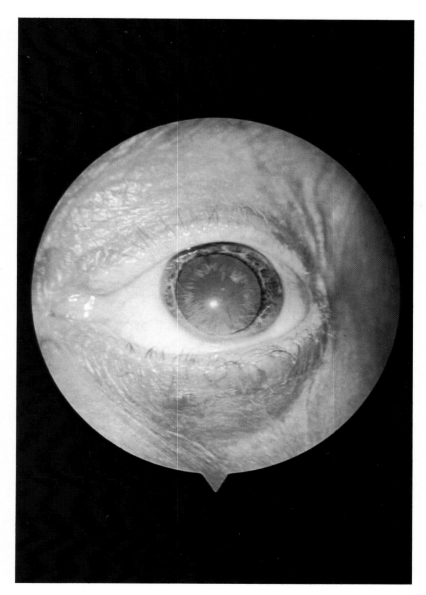

Fig. 43. Note a central lens opacity surrounded by clear lens through which the normal red reflex is seen. Clearly, interference to metabolism was operating when the innermost earliest fibres were being laid down; so this is a type of **congenital cataract.**

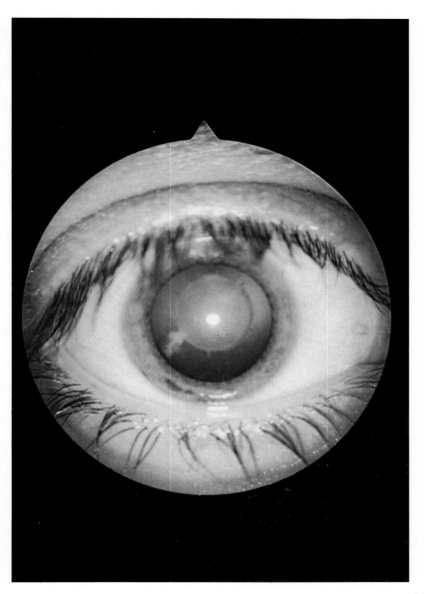

Fig. 44. A characteristic disc-shape loss of red reflex situated in the posterior part of the lens characteristic of **radiation cataract.**

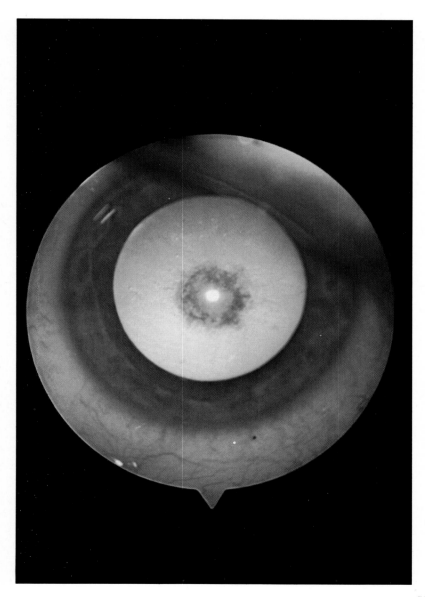

Fig. 45. A few globules seen adjacent to the highlight of the examiner's light caused by long continued use of systemic steroids, this is an early **steroid cataract.**

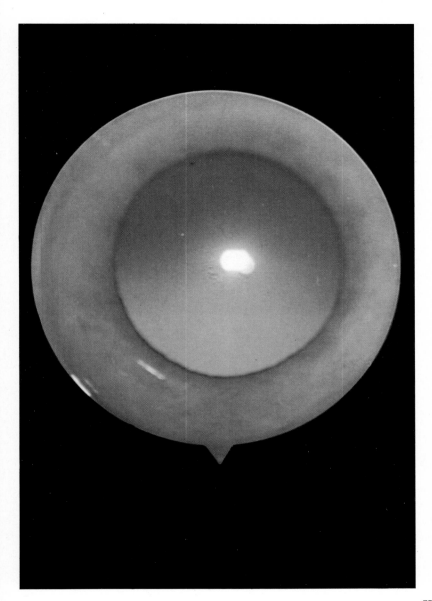

Fig. 46. Hypertensive retinopathy. Many patients with hypertension initially complain of visual changes, disregarding their other symptoms. There may be slight changes in visual acuity, the outside of the eyes may appear normal, but on the inside this fundus picture can be seen. Note the calibre and the crossing of the arteries over the veins. Haemorrhages may be seen but the main changes are arterial (see **figs. 47 & 52).**

Fig. 47. A florid hypertensive retinopathy. Note the arterial changes, *i.e.* the increased "silver wire" reflections from the arteries with marked A/V nipping.

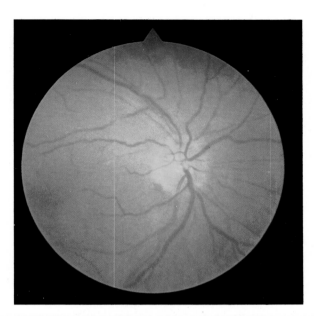

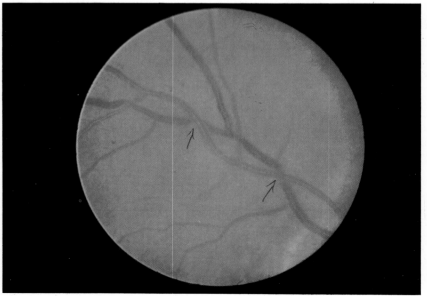

Fig. 48. A case of **diabetic retinopathy**. Note the vascular changes predominantly at the posterior pole of the eye with "dot and blot haemorrhages" and hard exudates arranged side by side. There are minimal arterio-venous changes.

Fig. 49. Many diseases, particularly the auto-immune or collagen systems, can show a retinopathy, and here is seen the retinopathy of lupus erythematosus. Notice the many soft white exudates.

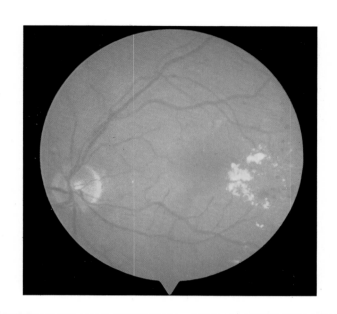

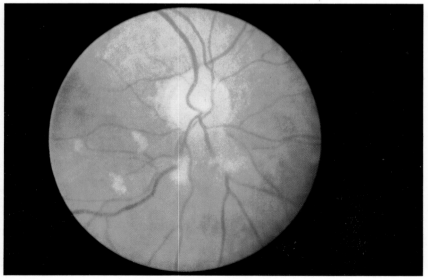

Fig. 50. Toxoplasmosis choroidoretinitis. These cases commonly present later with an active focus towards one edge of the lesion. Note the white scarring and the black proliferation of pigment; an area of active inflammation on this will present as an ill-defined whitish opacity, the area being white because it is thicker and thus less of the normal red reflex will be showing through. This is the most common cause of an acute focal choroidoretinitis.

Fig. 51. Patches of disseminated choroidoretinitis; that is, confluent rounded patches of scarring and proliferation of the pigment epithelium. Such a picture should immediately suggest syphilis.

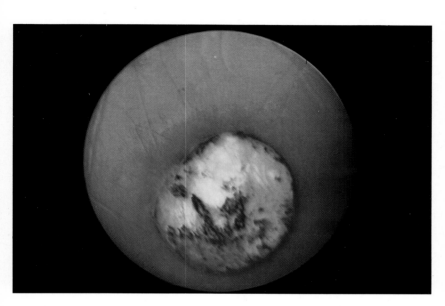

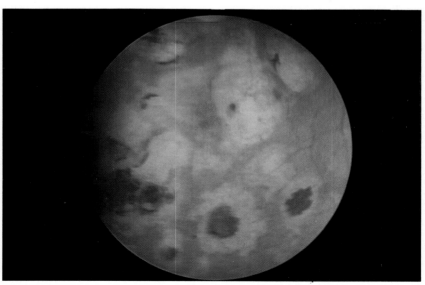

Fig. 52. Superimposed on a hypertensive retinopathy may be disc changes. Note the congested disc with the fine capillaries particularly on the nasal side with early swelling. This is early **papilloedema.**

Fig. 53. A further stage of papilloedema. Note the gross swelling of the disc and the way the vessels tumble over the edge. Apart from this, note that there is relatively little vascular change with no retinopathy. This is the sort of swelling seen in benign intercranial hypertension.

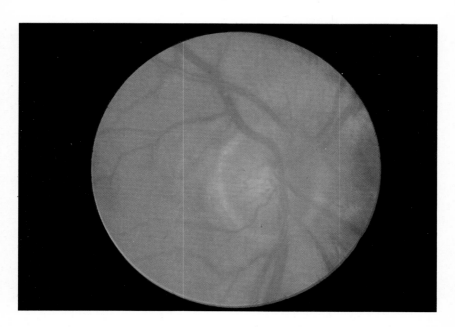

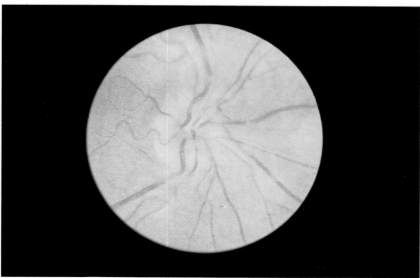

Fig. 54. A severe form of papilloedema. Note the obliterated disc margins, the gross swelling and the way the vessels tumble over the edge of the disc, the whole being surrounded by a ring of scattered haemorrhages. This gross sort of papilloedema may be seen in renal hypertension or in tumours of the optic nerve or of the brain.

Fig. 55. The early suspicious glaucomatous cup. Note that the cup is enlarged and the vessels dip over the edge. Such a disc, even in the absence of symptoms, should be referred for the assessments of **chronic glaucoma.** The visual acuity may be normal. This form of glaucoma (as opposed to acute glaucoma — the red eye) is insidious, there being no pain or redness; only a reduction of visual function extending over many months. The optic disc gives the clue.

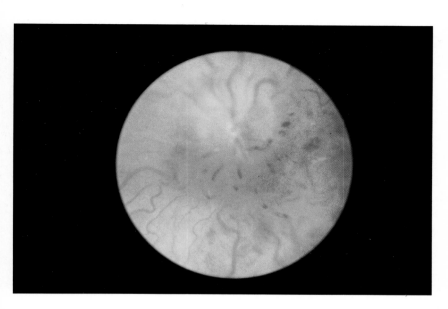

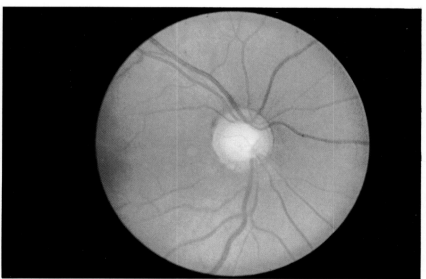

Fig. 56. The early glaucomatous field. Note that on the left is the right normal central field with the blind spot. On the right is seen the classical **arcuate scotoma** as the blind spot extends up and over the point of fixation. This is due to pressure on the optic nerve which presses on the normal physiological cup, enlarges it and pushes it out of the eye. Such pressure can lead to almost complete blindness if it continues for years.

Fig. 57. Optic atrophy. When a patient who is complaining of visual changes has normal physical signs at the front of the eye, but pale discs like this are noted, the fields should be examined by confrontation. Pituitary tumours, orbital tumours, the end result of disseminated sclerosis and spirochaetal disease may all present with similar optic atrophy.

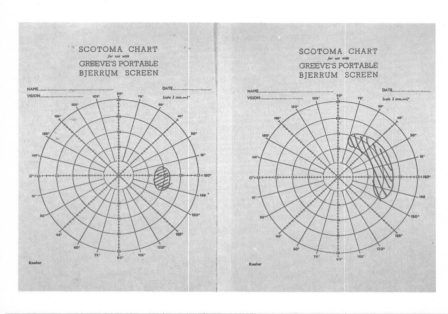

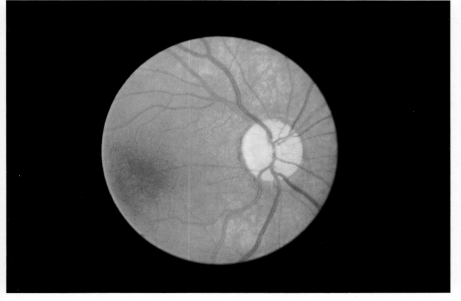

SUDDEN LOSS OF VISION

Fig. 58. Block of the central retinal artery (lower branch). This patient complains of sudden loss of vision. After the outside of the eye is examined and appears normal the inside shows this condition. Note the loss of red reflex below, there being a whitish colour. This is because the retina is thickened and less choroid shows through. The other important physical sign is that the artery is collapsed in that portion of the retina. The white area is thus a patch of ischaemic necrosis due to a block of the artery supplying it. Sometimes the whole retinal artery will be blocked so that the whole fundus presents this milky appearance and the ensuing visual loss is catastrophic and permanent. Causes are numerous but the one that should first be considered is **temporal or giant cell arteritis,** particularly in the elderly. If the condition is not diagnosed, the other eye may well be affected and the patient made permanently blind. Other causes are hypertension, arteriosclerosis, emboli, collagen diseases,

Fig. 59. Retinal vein thrombosis. The patient complains of a loss of vision but not as dramatic or as severe as in the previous case. The artery is still pumping blood into the eye and the obstruction may be partway along the vein (in this case the upper half) or sometimes at the disc. In either case the retina distal to the block is broken up by a sheet of haemorrhages extending from the point of obstruction.

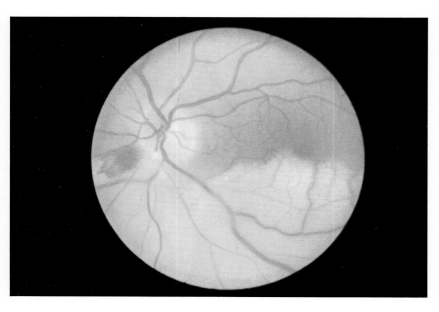

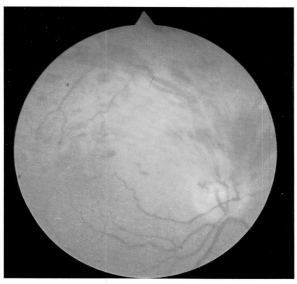

Fig. 60. A retinal detachment. This patient complains of sudden loss or change in vision, perhaps preceded by black spots or flashing lights. The retinal detachment is caused by a retinal hole; as the hole is forming the retina is irritated, giving flashing lights subjectively. The hole may tear across small capillaries giving a minor vitreous haemorrhage and these are seen as black flies or cobwebs by the patient. The retina then detaches and hangs into the eye as a grey balloon. Such a localised loss of red reflex with this characteristic greyness should immediately lead to diagnosis of a retinal detachment. Treatment is urgent and requires admission to hospital; otherwise the detachment will progress.

Fig. 61. A total retinal detachment in a patient who did not present himself until his visual loss had been almost complete. The detachment had become total and the retina can be seen against the back of the lens in folds. There is a complete loss of the red reflex.

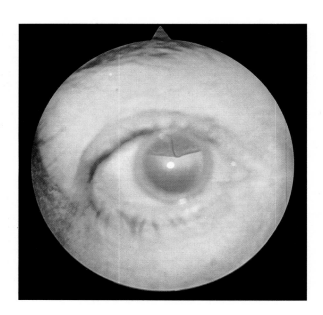

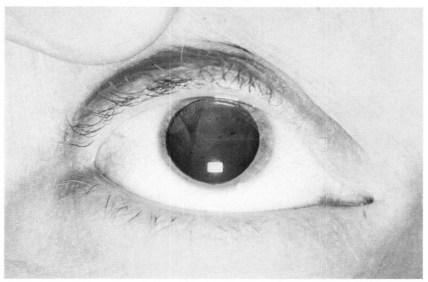

Part 4

Eye Injuries

MINOR EYE INJURIES are extremely common; they range from a superficial foreign body, traumatic ulcers, corrosive injuries to the "black eye". Unfortunately, some major eye injuries of the globe or orbit may appear superficially like a "black eye", while penetrating eye injuries may be completely misdiagnosed.

MINOR INJURIES:
CORNEAL FOREIGN BODIES

Fig. 62. This patient states that something has blown into his eye. The visual acuity may be normal but there may be a considerable amount of lacrimation or photophobia. The foreign body can be seen slightly off-centre below and to the left of the pupil immediately to the left of the large central highlight of the examiner's hand light. It must be removed and after anaesthetising the cornea an attempt should be made to sweep it off with some cotton wool wrapped round an orange stick or a match stick.

Fig. 63. Here an attempt is being made to sweep the foreign body off; but it is often unsuccessful.

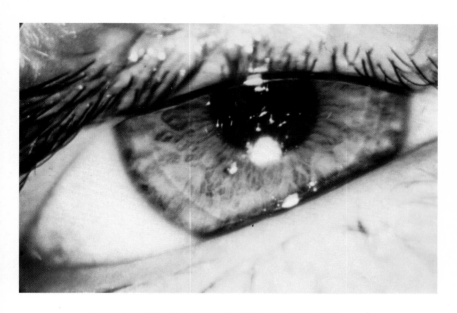

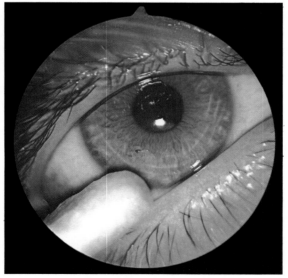

Fig. 64. The classical eye instrument for removing the corneal foreign body is a corneal spud. Here it is in use on an anaesthetised eye. As can be seen, it is flat but not sharp and therefore cannot do any untoward damage to the eye should the doctor or patient move involuntarily. The end is placed under the foreign body and it is flicked off the cornea.

Fig. 65. The three instruments which may be used· for removal of a foreign body. Uppermost is the classical corneal spud which is easily used by those not experienced in ophthalmology – but is rather unwieldy and will give a certain amount of superficial damage. Below that is the knife needle favoured by eye surgeons. This is extremely sharp and if used in unskilled hands can be thrust through the cornea. Below that is a commercially available orange stick with cotton wool wrapped around each end. These are ideal for attempting to sweep off a corneal foreign body. Below these two are the close-ups of the eye instruments themselves. Whichever way is used to remove the foreign body, some epithelium must be lost as well, so that fluorescein must be placed in the eye to estimate the loss of epithelium.

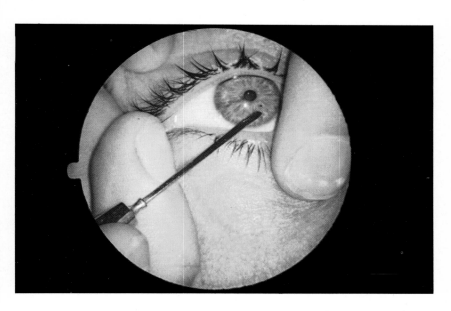

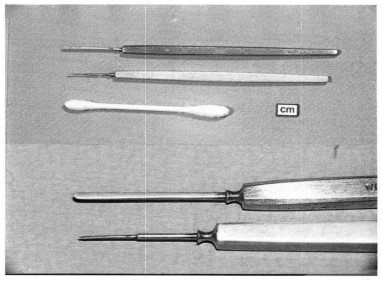

Fig. 66. Note the small green area at the site of the foreign body (same case as **fig. 62**). The green area is pathognomonic of a **corneal ulcer** and all corneal ulcers should have the eye covered.

Fig. 67. If a metallic foreign body has been in for more than a few hours as it has been resting on a liquid medium it will rust and when it is removed a **rust ring** will remain behind. Note the round circular brown ring which is within the substance of the cornea – not on it. The removal of this will probably require expert assistance.

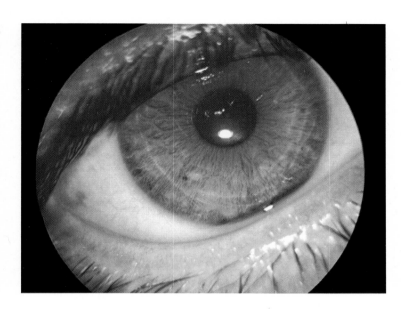

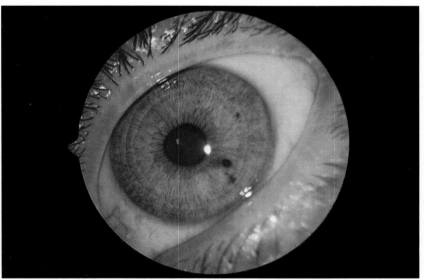

SUBTARSAL FOREIGN BODY

Fig. 68. This patient complains of something in his eye. Careful examination shows the absence of a corneal foreign body or a foreign body in the lower or lateral fornices. In this type of case the lid should be everted as described in the method of examination. Here is seen the classical appearance of a foreign body in this situation. It should be removed with cotton wool or a handkerchief and the cornea subsequently stained with fluorescein to show any ulcer present.

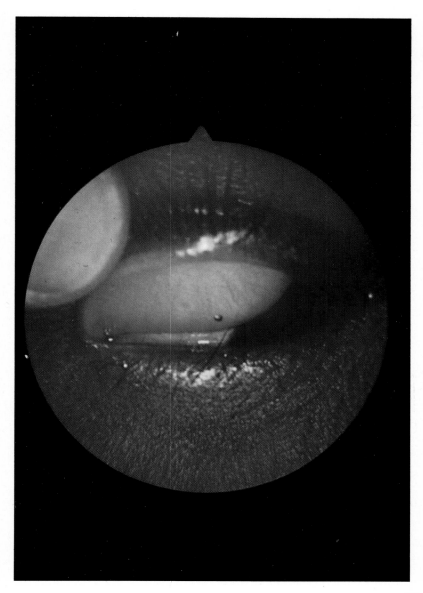

CORNEAL ULCERS

Fig. 69. A **traumatic corneal ulcer.** This patient complains of something in his eye. Examination should be done in this order:

(1) Is there a corneal foreign body?

(2) Is there a subtarsal foreign body?

(3) If not, has the foreign body gone onto the eye, scratched it and come off again? Fluorescein will show this.

The eye should be covered with a pad and bandage to facilitate healing.

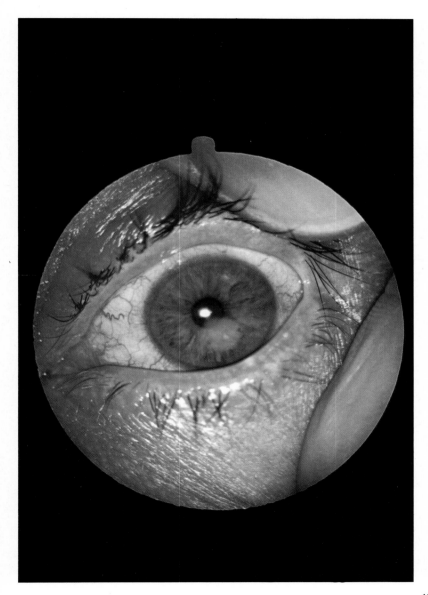

Fig. 70. Burns with hot solid material should be assessed as in **fig. 69.** Fluorescein shows not only typical green areas of ulceration but white coagulated material beneath them. These cases are best referred for specialist attention.

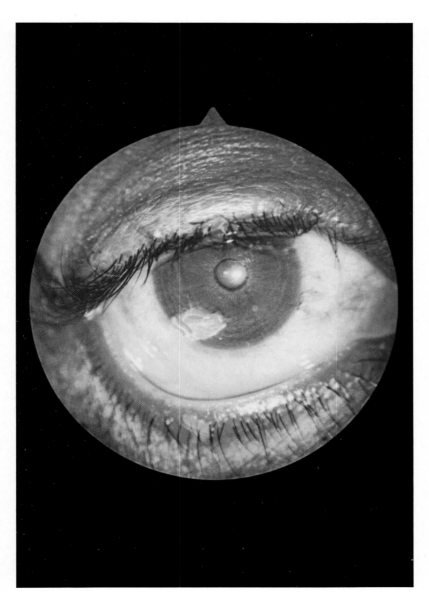

Fig. 71. Corrosive burns due to ammonia as in this case are diagnosed by fluorescein and then referred for specialist treatment. If the raw areas on the cornea and conjunctiva are opposite similar raw areas on the back of the lids the two may fuse together. Treatment is immediate lavage with copious amounts of water. Do not wait for suitable neutralising agents, but plunge the patient's head under a tap or into a fire bucket, or any other nearby source of water.

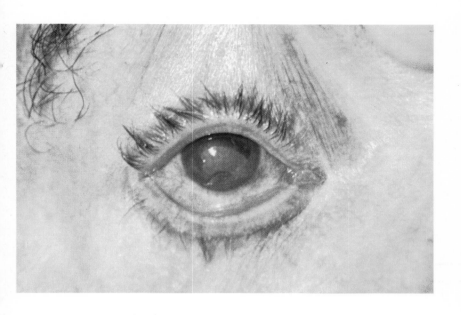

"BLACK EYES"

Fig. 72. This is the typical **"black eye"** which can be defined as a lid haematoma. It is classically caused by a blunt injury to the orbit. However, all cases of a black eye should be assessed with two things in mind:

(1) Is the eye intact? Has there been a concussion injury to the eye? See **figs. 74 - 80;**

(2) Has there been a concussion injury to the orbit? See **figs. 81 - 83.**

In such a case as depicted here it may be impossible to see the eye, but in a surprisingly short time the swelling will regress.

Fig. 73. A black eye after the swelling has regressed. Note the haematoma of the lid and the sub-conjunctival haemorrhage, but note also that the cornea is bright and the pupil is round and central with a red reflex showing through. Clearly there is no intra-ocular damage.

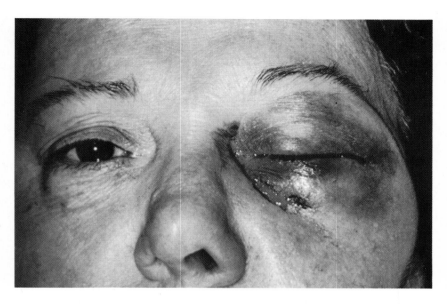

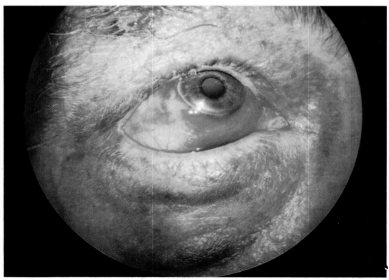

MAJOR EYE INJURIES (CLOSED)

Fig. 74. Blood in the anterior chamber or a **hyphaema**. This classically follows a contusion injury to the eye and may present with the external physical signs of a black eye. Note that the blood is floating around in the anterior chamber and a level can be seen below. These will be the physical signs seen recently after the injury.

Fig. 75. A classical hyphaema after the blood has been allowed to settle. There is an associated traumatic dilation of the pupil (mydriasis). In these cases the eye has received a severe injury which takes it out of the category of a simple black eye into the category of a severe eye injury.

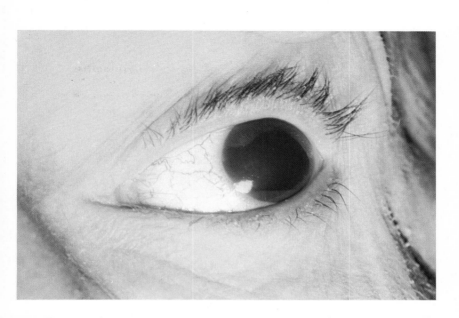

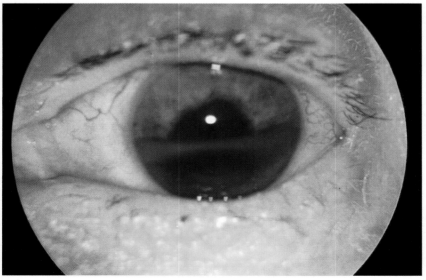

Fig. 76. Rupture of the globe. The blow here has given a hyphaema and has split the coats of the eye concentric with the limbus as shown by the dark swelling to one side. This again is obviously a severe injury.

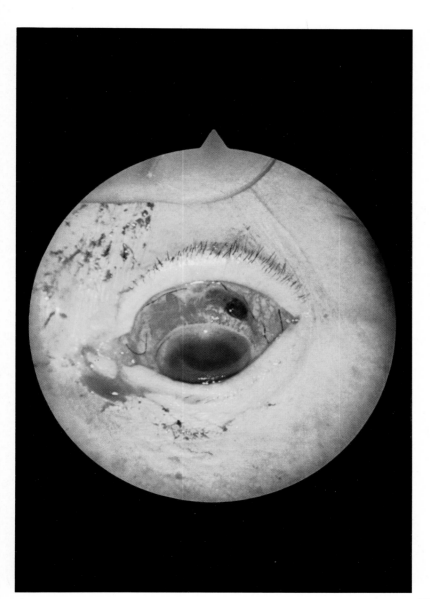

Fig. 77. In this case the pressure wave generated by the blow on the front of the eye has passed from the back of the cornea and struck the iris, perhaps giving a hyphaema in the early stage, but also has caused a tear of the root of the iris from its insertion, a so-called **iridodialysis.**

Fig. 78. Concussion cataract and injury to the iris caused by a blow on the eye, the pressure wave striking the iris and the lens.

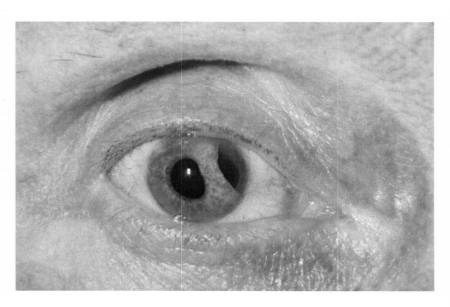

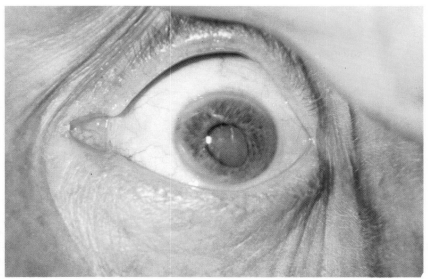

Fig. 79. Oedema of the retina with **commotio retinae.** This may present as a simple black eye; the front of the eye appears clear, but at the back of the eye can be seen loss of red reflex around the inferior temporal vessels. Note the patch of white speckling which may in severe cases become confluent. The white areas are due to retinal thickening caused by the blow on the front of the eye.

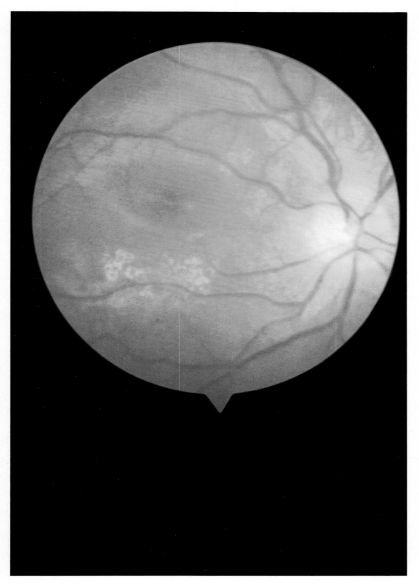

Fig. 80. Choroidal rupture. In these cases the pressure wave is greater than in previous ones and it strikes the back of the eye, severing the retina and the choroid. There may be retinal haemorrhages as seen here, the white areas being the splits in choroid with the sclera showing through.

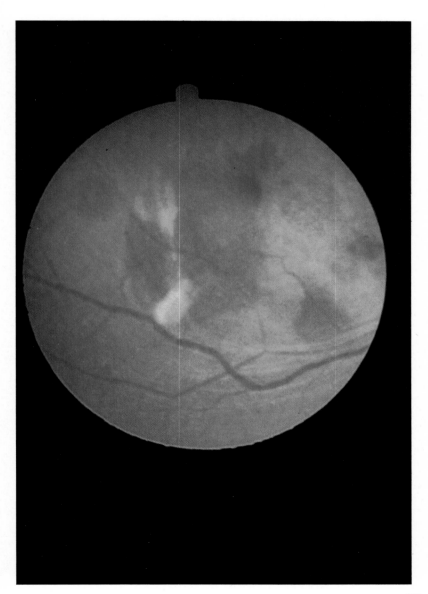

MAJOR ORBITAL INJURIES

Fig. 81. Blow-out fracture of the orbit. These cases may appear also as simple black eyes and may have any of the contusion injuries of the globe itself. The pressure wave generated within the orbit strikes the orbital walls and fractures this through where it is weakest and most unsupported, *i.e.* the floor (the roof of the maxillary sinus). A variable quantity of the contents of the lower part of the orbit is incarcerated in the roof of the maxillary sinus. There is thus:

(1) Enophthalmos;
(2) Anaesthesia of the infra-orbital nerve;
(3) Vertical double vision.

Fig. 82. The patient is now attempting to look up. Notice that the gap between the lids and the limbus is greater on the left eye than the right, *i.e.* the right eye is not moving up as the muscles are incarcerated in the fracture of the floor of the orbit.

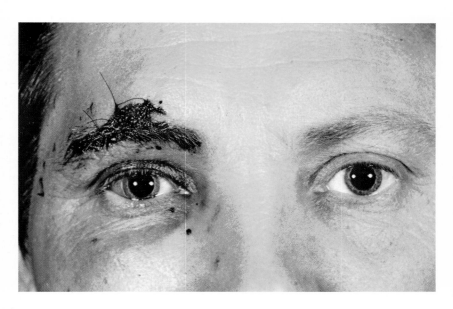

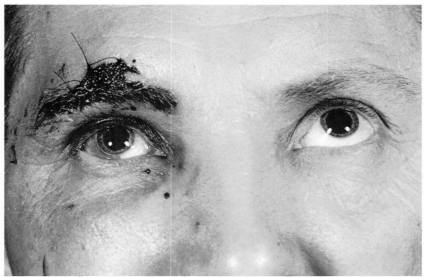

Fig. 83. X-ray to show the little hernial sac, *i.e.* some of the contents of the orbit displaced down in the maxillary antrum. Thus all cases of a black eye should be examined not only for injury to the eye but also to the integrity of the orbit as well.

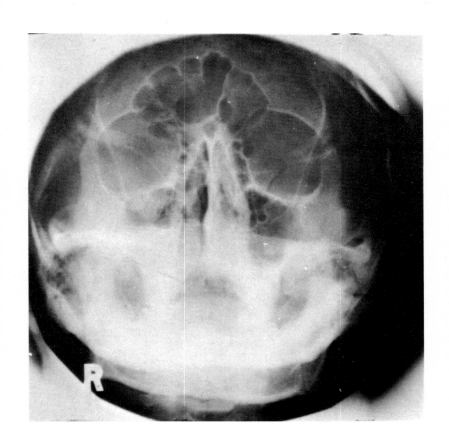

MAJOR EYE INJURIES (OPEN)

Fig. 84. Penetrating eye injury. The patient classically states one of two things: *(a)* he was using a hammer and chisel on concrete, or *(b)* using a grindstone without goggles. In each case a small piece of metal flies backwards perhaps travelling at several hundred miles an hour, and passes into the eye. As the coats of the eye are severed, and as the pressure inside the eye is higher than that of the atmosphere, there is a tendency for the intra-ocular contents to prolapse. If the penetration is anterior this is characterised by an **iris prolapse** which is the knuckle of pigment seen on the side of the limbus associated with **distortion of the pupil** as some of the iris forming the border of the pupil is outside the eye. Such cases should be admitted immediately, as anything that raises the intra-ocular pressure may prolapse further eye contents.

Fig. 85. Traumatic cataract. The foreign body may strike the lens, rendering it opaque within a matter of hours. This makes subsequent visualisation and removal very difficult.

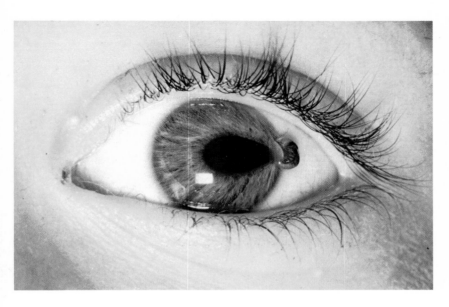

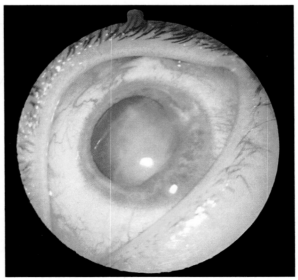

Fig. 86. Multiple lacerations of the face and lids. These are very common with windscreen injuries and bottle fights. Such cases should be examined carefully, particularly in respect of the lacerations involving the lid margins. If they are involved they are probably best sutured by an eye surgeon, particularly those on the medial side, as they may well have involved the lower canaliculus — in which case immediate surgery is needed. All these cases should be examined for lacerations of the globe.

Fig. 87. The same case as the preceding one. When the swelling had reduced, it was possible to examine the globe carefully: a doubtful area on the temporal side can be seen.

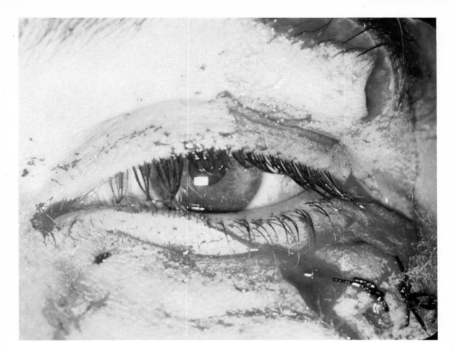

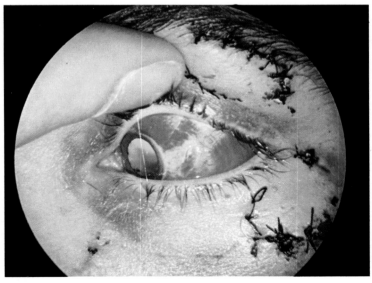

Fig. 88. Close-up of the doubtful area in fig. 87 which shows an obvious full-thickness laceration requiring urgent attention.

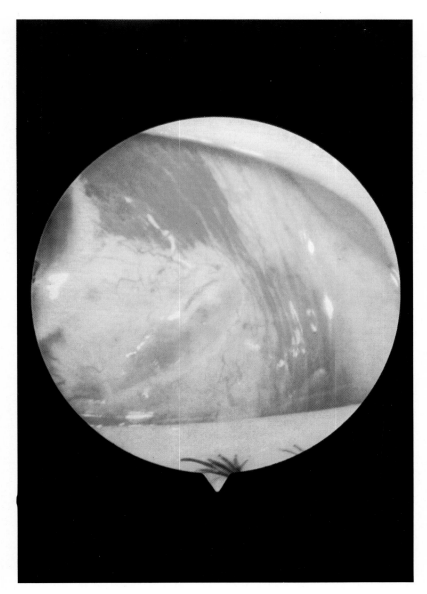

Part 5

Miscellaneous

A This section includes common clinical conditions that do not otherwise fit into the clinical patterns previously described.

B After the conditions noted above there follows another collection of miscellaneous pathological processes of less importance but all of which show clear physical signs which are characteristic of their conditions and which can be easily seen by employing the method of examination detailed previously.

(A) ABNORMALITIES OF LID POSITION

Fig. 89. Note that this patient has a normal lid aperture on her left side as shown by the limbus touching the lower lid and overlapped by the upper one. Compare this with the aperture on the other side. Note that the limbus is separated from both lids by a white margin, thus in the upper lid there is **lid retraction** and by the lower lid the eye is obviously **pushed forwards.** This combination of lid retraction and/or proptosis can be very misleading.

Fig. 90. A case of **thyrotoxicosis,** but note that there is bilateral symmetrical lid retraction and no proptosis, *i.e.* the limbus is just touched by the lower lids but there is a gap above.

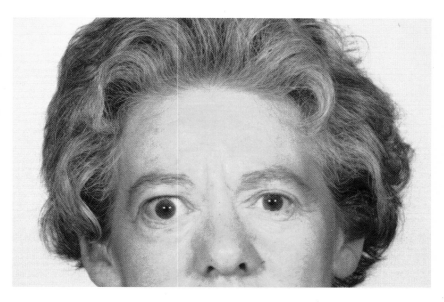

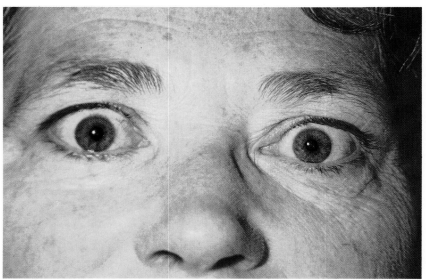

Fig. 91. A case of bilateral symmetrical lid retraction and proptosis, *i.e.* gap between the limbus and lid above and below.

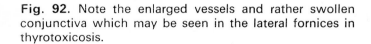

Fig. 92. Note the enlarged vessels and rather swollen conjunctiva which may be seen in the lateral fornices in thyrotoxicosis.

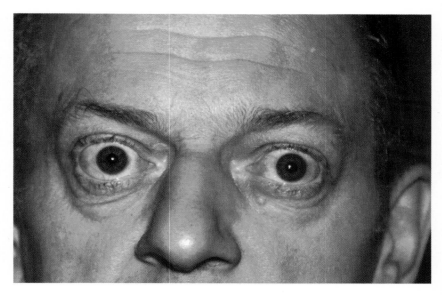

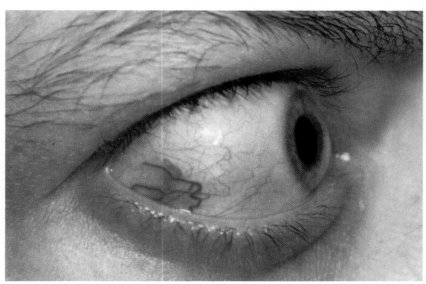

Fig. 93. A case of bilateral symmetrical proptosis, *i.e.* gap present between the limbus and the lower lids but no lid retraction.

Fig. 94. Entropion. The patient complains of a sore, running, red eye. On first examination conjunctivitis may be suspected, but a closer look shows that the lower lid is rolled over and the lashes are rubbing the eye. It is no use treating this condition with eye drops. The patient must be referred for minor surgery to turn the lid over. This is a condition very commonly seen in old people.

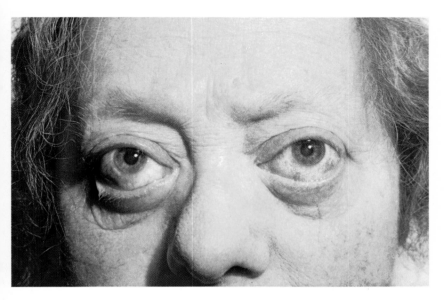

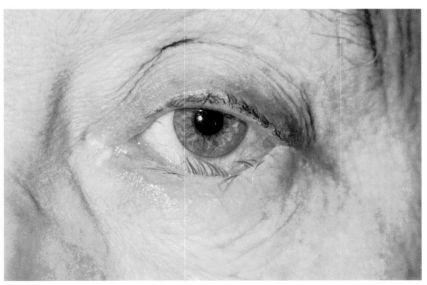

Fig. 95. Entropion. A case similar to **fig. 94,** but less obvious.

Fig. 96. Ectropion. In these old people the lower lid loses its tone and drops away from the globe, particularly on the medial side. In these cases they complain of a running eye as tears cannot drain down the passages. The primary cause is the lid position and this must be treated to restore continuity of the tear flow and drainage.

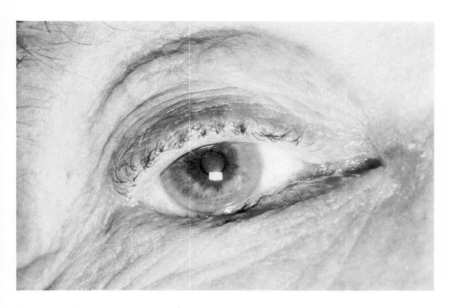

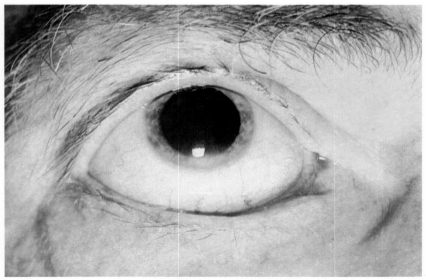

Fig. 97. Ectropion. Another case showing how easily the condition can be missed. Note that the lower lid has fallen slightly away from the globe on the inner side.

Fig. 98. Ectropion. Severe ectropion caused by a tumour of the centre of the lid.

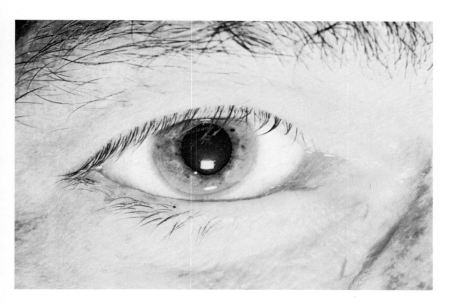

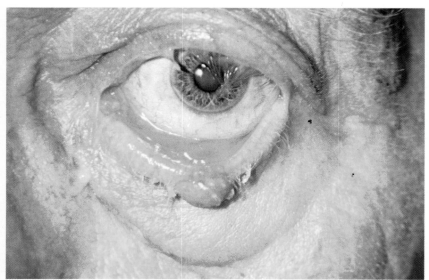

PATHOLOGY OF THE LIDS

Fig. 99. Stye. The patient complains of a sore, swollen lid of a few days duration. On examination there is a tender inflammatory swelling; on close inspection it is seen to be pointing round a lash follicle. Thus a stye can be defined as an acute infective process involving the lash follicles. It should be encouraged to point with "hot spoon bathings" and an antibiotic ointment to prevent a secondary conjunctivitis. Once it has pointed the offending lash should be removed.

Fig. 100. Infected Meibomian cyst. This patient also presents with a sore swollen eyelid; it is infective, but close inspection shows that it is not pointing around the lashes, *i.e.* it is not a stye, but above the lash line at the junction of the inner and middle thirds in this case. It should be treated along the same lines as a stye, but the patient should be told that once it has settled there will be a residual nodule present which will almost certainly need incision and curettage.

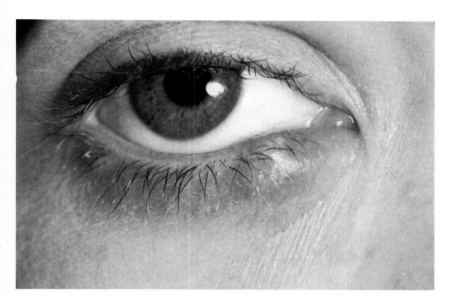

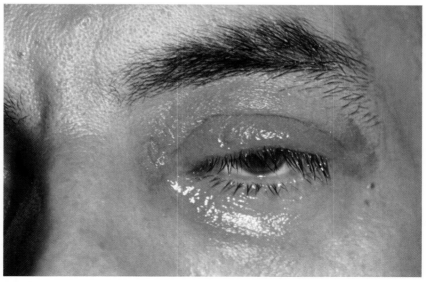

Fig. 101. A **Meibomian cyst** which may or may not become infected like the previous figure in which case it may be confused with a stye.

Fig. 102. Two **Meibomian cysts** which are granulations on the glands of the deep surface of the lids. They may be seen by everting the appropriate lid.

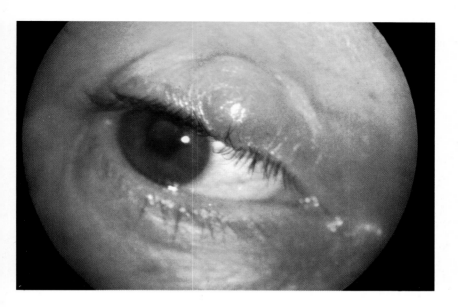

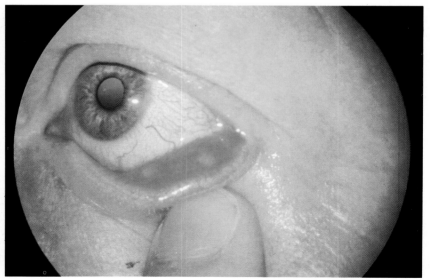

Fig. 103. A **basal cell carcinoma** or rodent ulcer. These are extremely common around the eyes. The diagnosis is made by the presence of a raised, pearly nodule perhaps with a central ulcer. They are difficult to treat because either surgery or radiotherapy may give untoward complications.

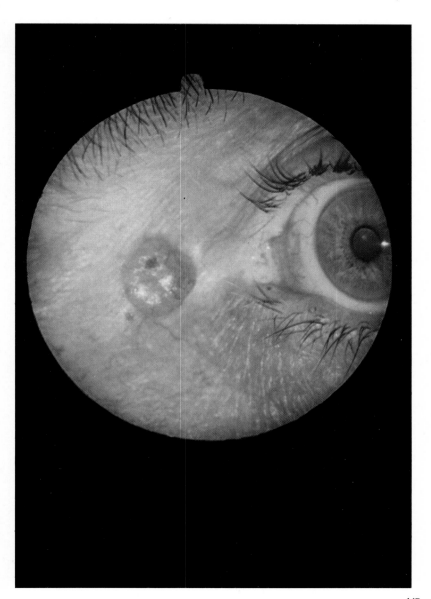

MUSCLE PATHOLOGY

Fig. 104. Squint. A squint may be defined as a loss of parallelism of the visual axis. Ocular posture is a **reflex action,** thus any interference with this reflex may give a squint. Thus a **sensory defect** — *e.g.* a corneal scar, a uniocular congenital cataract or a uniocular retinal affliction — may give a squint because there is no stimulus to keep the eye straight. Similarly a **loss of the central fusion sense,** as is common in mentally deficient children, may also give a squint. Interference on the **motor side,** that is a nerve palsy or a neuromuscular abnormality; or a congenital abnormality of the muscles themselves may give a squint. In most ordinary cases the child is far-sighted and has to over-focus for distance and consequently while giving excessive accommodation for, say, reading also shows excessive convergence and turns one eye in. The danger is that the eye turned in may be suppressed and there may be a permanent loss of vision. Because of this, all squints should be seen promptly as early treatment may restore binocular vision and because in rare cases there may be some disease causing the ocular deviation.

STRABISMUS

(A) ESTROPIA
     1. Non-paralytic (comitant)
        a. Non-accommodative.
        b. Accommodative.
        c. Combined accommodative + non-accommodative
     2. Paretic (non-comitant)

(B) EXOTROPIA
     1. Intermittent
     2. Constant

(C) HYPERTROPIA
     1. Paralytic
     2. Non-Paralytic

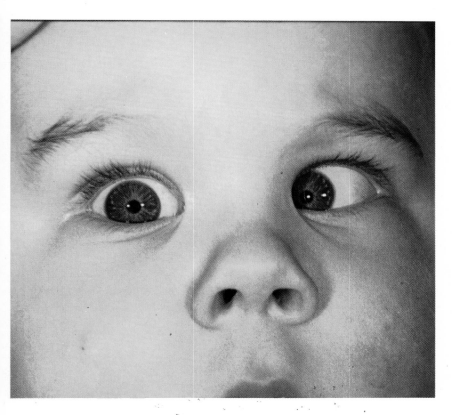

(L) ESOTROPIA

DISORDERS OF THE TEARS

Fig. 105. Epiphora, or a running eye. Diagram of the left tear passages showing that the tears may pass out over the globe, downwards and medially through the canaliculi into the lacrimal sac, through the lacrimal passages and into the nose. There are two occasions in life when epiphora can occur. In a **newborn child;** the flap of membrane at the lower part of the tear passages does not canalise and the tears are dammed up. The baby has a continuously running eye which intermittently gets infected. Treatment is massage of the tear sac against the nasal bones when in many cases the pressure may force the flap open. If this not effective, a probing may be needed.

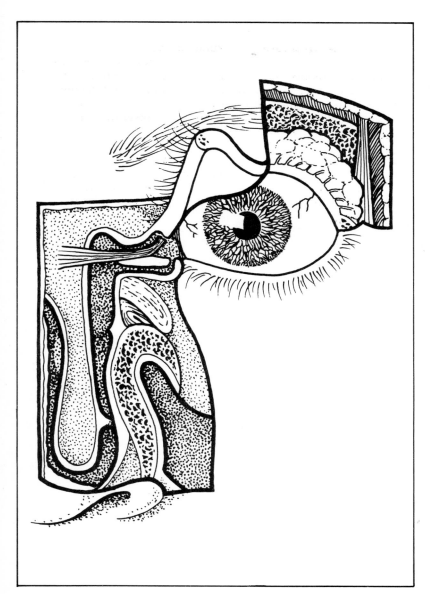

Fig. 106. In adults there is a chronic inflammatory stricture of the lower end of the tear sac and this may give an intermittent swelling near the inner canthus as seen here, with a running eye.

Fig. 107. An **abscess of the lacrimal sac** due to infection of the stagnating tear sac contents (same case as **fig. 106**). Such cases are best referred for surgery.

Dacryocytadenitis

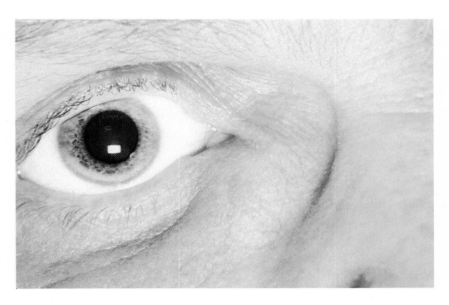

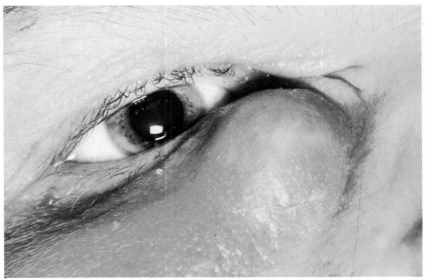

ALLERGY

Fig. 108. Allergy. This is becoming increasingly common and is particularly associated with Penicillin or Neomycin and sometimes drops used in the treatment of glaucoma. The diagnosis is made with the appearance of a red eye with eczematous skin changes as seen here. Clearly the drops must be stopped, but this may be difficult if the patient requires them for treatment of glaucoma. Such cases should be referred back to the eye surgeon.

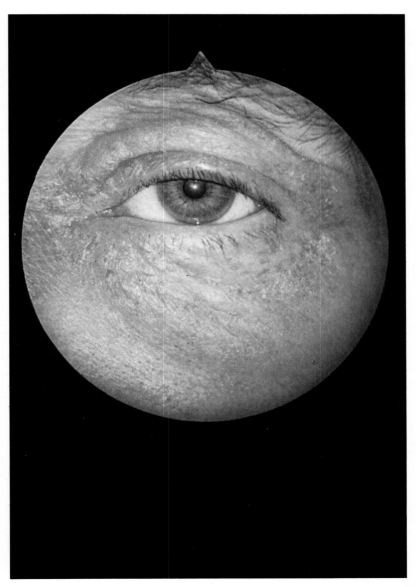

(B) LESS COMMON MISCELLANEOUS CONDITIONS

Fig. 109. Xanthelasma, showing the characteristic raised yellowish nodules situated within the skin. They may be larger and indeed confluent around the upper and lower lids of both eyes. They are said to indicate the presence of diabetes.

Fig. 110. A **lateral tarsorrhaphy.** Note that the lids have been sutured together some time previously and the sutures removed. This manoeuvre is employed in all cases where corneal cover is deficient, *i.e.* thyroid disease, any form of proptosis, VIIth nerve palsy, etc.

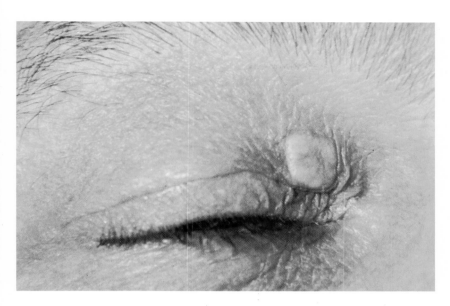

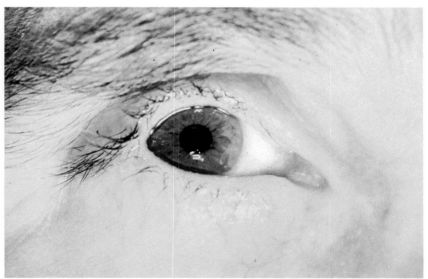

Fig. 111. Conjunctiva of the upper fornix. Note **mascara deposited sub-conjunctivally.** The upper lid has been everted and along its edge may be seen sub-conjunctival black patches which are due to the deposition of mascara which has been used for cosmetic purposes over some years. This condition is becoming increasingly common.

Fig. 112. Vernal catarrh. The patient is usually young and complains of symptoms suggestive of conjunctivits, but itching is a prominent symptom.

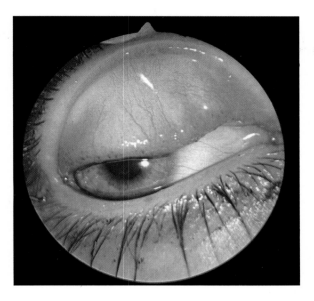

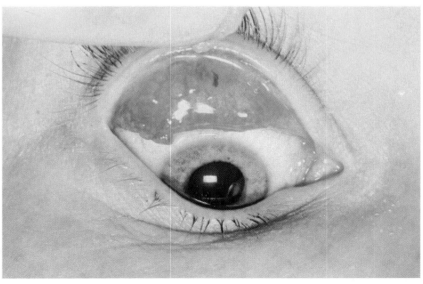

Fig. 113. Argyrosis. This condition results from the deposition of silver from the long continued use of silver nitrate drops over many years.

Fig. 114. A spontaneous **sub-conjunctival haemorrhage.** These are common in middle-aged and elderly people and an isolated episode is of no significance. Further attacks may mean that there is a bleeding diathesis present.

_— ↑ B.P._
— bleeding diathesis
— straining — lifting
_— B.M_
& etc.

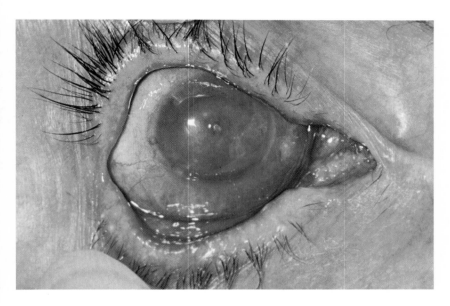

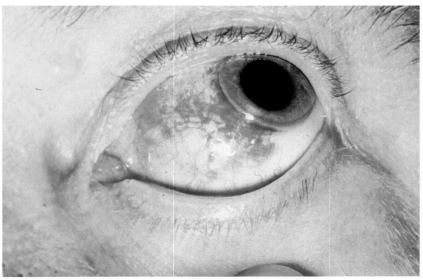

Fig. 115. A patch of sc̲l̲e̲r̲i̲t̲i̲s̲. Note that the conjunctival congestion is only localised, but that there are also deeper vessels involved. Such a condition may be associated with systemic diseases particularly of the arthritic type.

Fig. 116. Scleromalacia. This is thinning of the sclera due to recurrent attacks of scleritis (see figure above.)

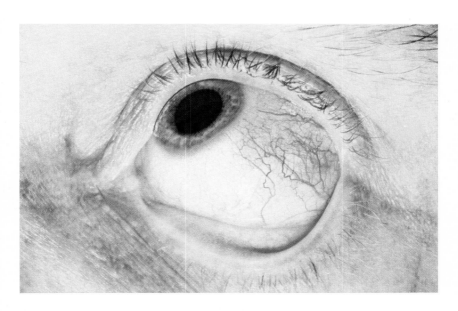

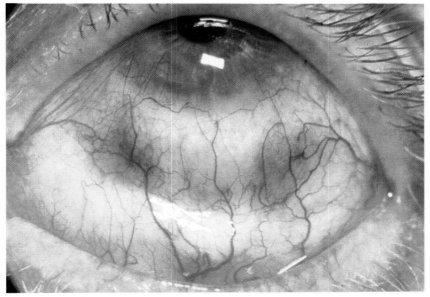

Fig. 117. A **carotico-cavernous sinus fistula.** The back pressure produces this tremendous dilation and congestion of the conjunctival veins which is pathognomonic. In due course this congestion gives rise to raised intra-ocular pressure and the eye goes blind.

Fig. 118. A **pterygium.** This is an extremely common fibro-vascular membrane which may grow over the centre of the cornea. If it does so, it should be removed, as it may impede vision.

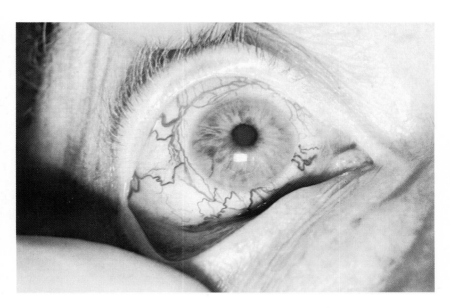

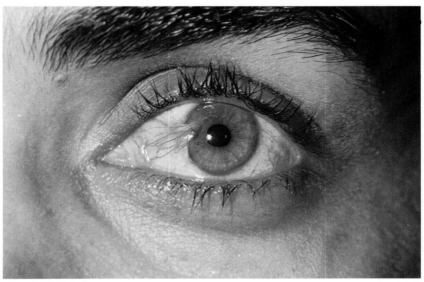

Fig. 119. A **dermoid tumour,** seen in its characteristic position straddling the limbus. It is yellowish and raised. It should be removed.

Fig. 120. A conjunctival **papilloma.** These may become very large and pedunculated, in which case they should be excised. They can be caused by a viral infection, in which case they may be multiple and extremely difficult to treat.

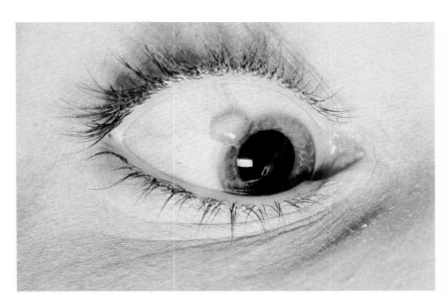

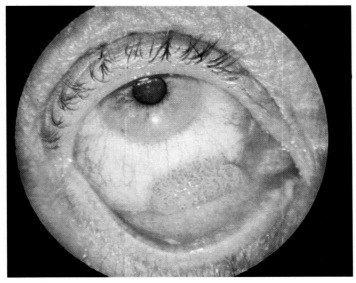

Fig. 121. An **arcus senilis.** This is a deposition of fat just within the limbus within the substance of the cornea. It is very common in middle-aged and old people and is of no significance.

Fig. 122. A **mustard gas keratitis.** This is usually bilateral, can be associated with much scarring and is characterised by the intra-corneal haemorrhages seen.

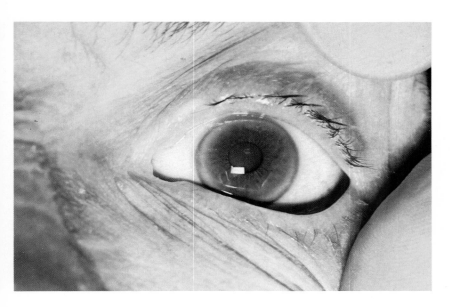

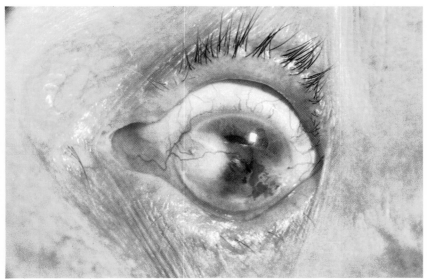

Fig. 123. A **failed corneal graft** because of a host-donor reaction. The circular scar at the bed of the donor may be seen together with the stitch marks and the haze involving both.

Fig. 124. A micro-corneal **contact lens**. The curved border of the lens can be seen slightly offset from the limbus. There are white fibrous patches behind an irregular pupil as this is a case of traumatic cataract which has been partially removed in a young person. Binocular vision can be given only by a contact lens or in some hands an intra-ocular plastic lens.

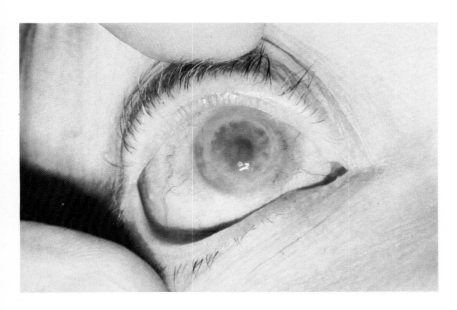

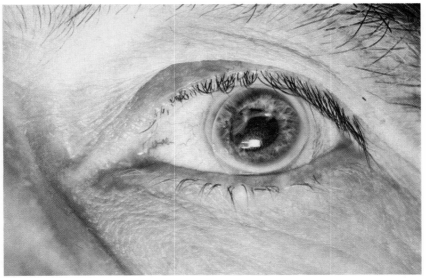

Fig. 125. The larger type of **contact lens** which fits on the eye, held in the patient's hand before insertion.

Fig. 126. The larger lens in position. Its rim can be seen well down in the fornix behind the lower lid with the ventilation hole at the limbus.

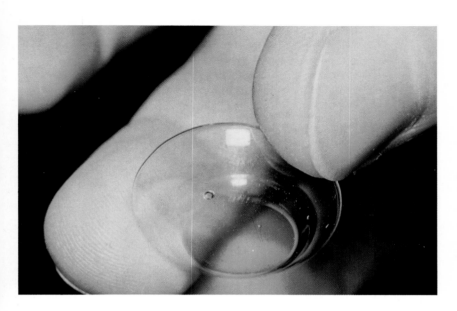

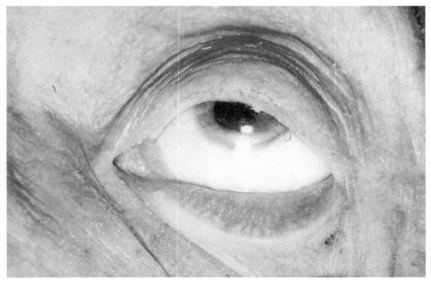

Fig. 127. An **intra-ocular plastic lens** can be seen in the anterior chamber. It has three limbs, two of which can be seen: one pointing outwards, the other downwards. This is also a case of a traumatic cataract and two small holes in the iris can be seen.

Fig. 128. An **aphakic eye,** *i.e.* one that has had the cataract removed showing the common surgical end result. Note that there is a clear black pupil and a small black segment at the periphery of the iris which is an iridectomy, a manoeuvre always done when the lens is being removed surgically.

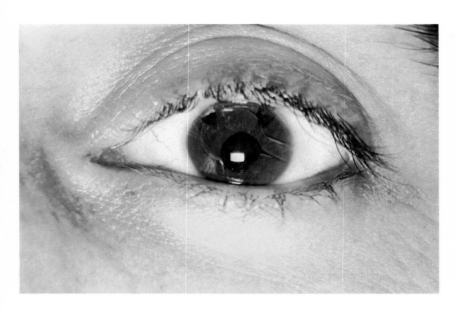

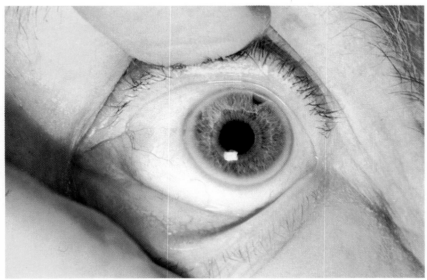

Fig. 129. An **after-cataract.** Older techniques of cataract removal meant leaving behind the capsule of the lens which occasionally thickened, giving an appearance like this. In these cases vision can only be restored by further minor operation.

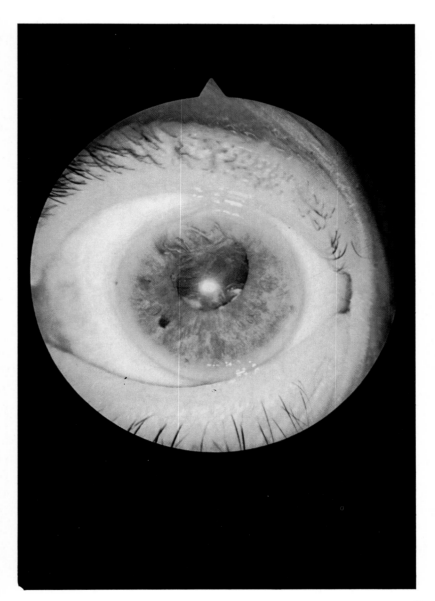

Fig. 130. **Rubeosis of the iris** in a diabetic. Note the pupil is off-centre, the iris atrophic and covered by a sheet of fine blood vessels. This is often the end result of diabetes affecting the eye.

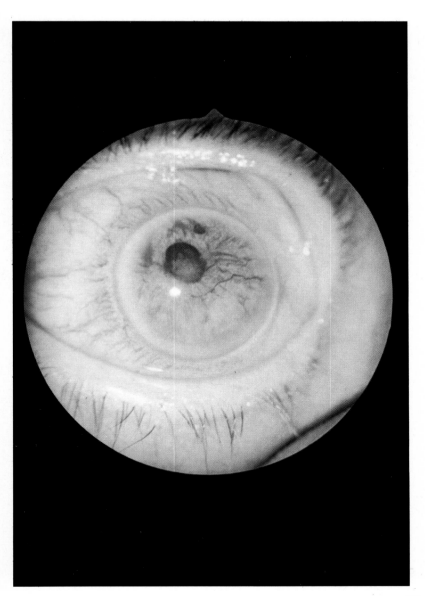

Fig. 131. Coloboma of the iris. Note that the iris is deficient downwards. This is a congenital defect because of faulty closure of the optic vesicle. It is frequently associated with similar defects in the retina and choroid. (See **fig. 134.**)

Fig. 132. A **malignant melanoma** of the iris and ciliary body. Note that there is a dark swelling pushing forward from the iris and is clearly arising from its root. Such a tumour, if left, will spread round the angle of the eye and give a form of glaucoma.

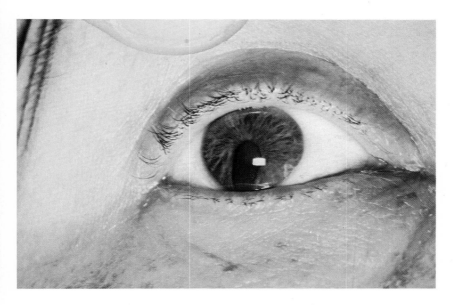

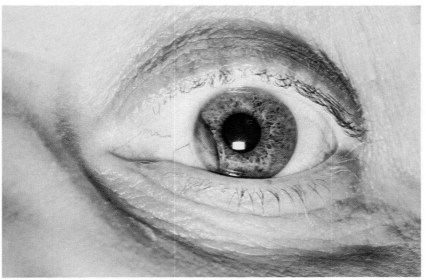

Fig. 133. An **endophthalmitis.** Note that the eye is congested, the pupil irregular due to iridocyclitis and there is a yellowish reflex (pus) from the back. This may be seen in cases of septacaemia when the eye virtually becomes a bag of pus.

Fig. 134. A **choroidal coloboma.** This is a congenital malformation of the choroid and retina often seen with an iris coloboma (see **fig. 131**). The normal retina and choroid is seen on one side while in the pale area is a deficiency of these structures, the ophthalmoscope viewing the sclera directly.

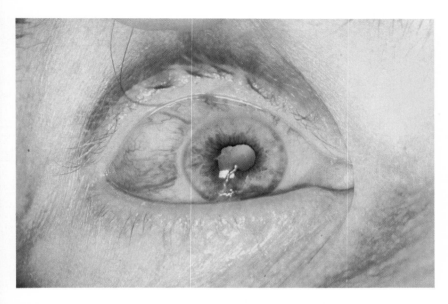

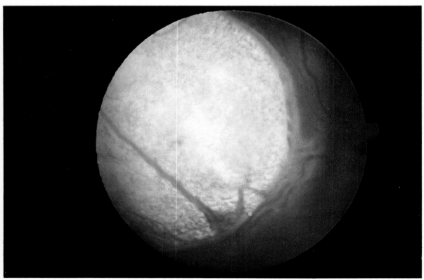

Fig. 135. A squint. Note that the left eye of the patient is convergent but that there is also a white reflex. This is pathognomonic of a **retinoblastoma** – a tumour which may be hereditary and perhaps involving both eyes of a child. (Compare with **fig. 104.**)

Fig. 136. A naevus of the choroid. A darkly pigmented patch occurring at the back of the eye. These require continued observation as they may become malignant and give rise to a malignant melanoma of the choroid.

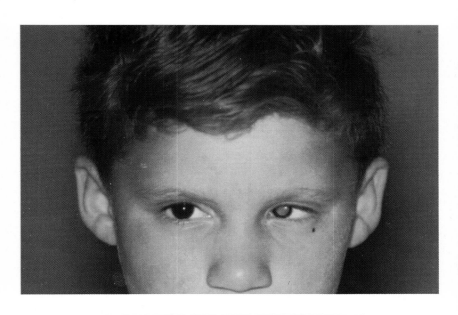

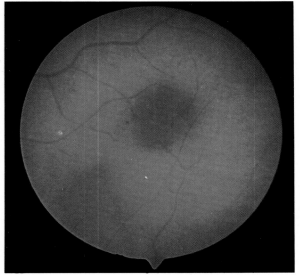

Fig. 137. Metastasis in the choroid. Two ill-defined yellow, slightly raised patches occurring in the eye of a woman dying from metastases. These are frequently larger and are probably more common than is suspected.

Fig. 138. Retinal folds. These can be seen traversing the back of the eye, spreading from the optic disc across the macula. In many cases they are due to pressure outside the eye by a tumour, or, rarely, in thyroid disease.

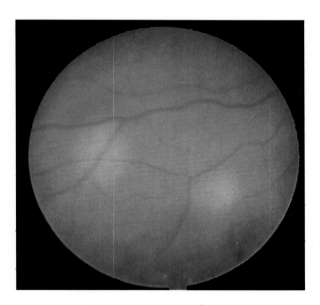

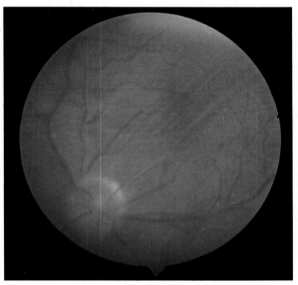

Acknowledgements

I TOOK MOST of these photographs with a Rayner Wray close-up camera for the external views, and a Kowa camera for the fundus. However, colleagues have been extremely kind in giving me some of their own photographs — in particular my friend and associate Mr. Peter MacFaul and my registrar at Bart's, Mrs. Enid Taylor. Mr. Tredinnick and Mr. Peter Cull of the Department of Medical Illustration of St. Bartholomew's Hospital were responsible for the majority of the external photographs in Part 1, and several other diagrams. Many eye house-surgeons at Bart's have helped find the clinical material. Finally, my sincere thanks to my secretary Miss Wendy Taylor, who welded the fractions into a composite whole.

M. A. BEDFORD
1971

Index